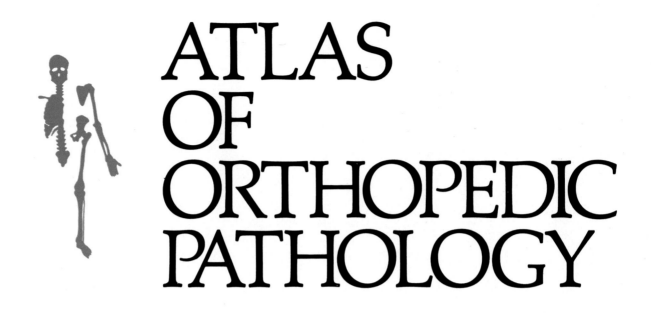

# ATLAS OF ORTHOPEDIC PATHOLOGY

# ATLASES IN
# DIAGNOSTIC SURGICAL PATHOLOGY

*Consulting Editor:*
**Gerald M. Bordin, M.D.**
Department of Pathology
Scripps Clinic and Research Foundation

*Forthcoming Titles:*

Colby and Lombard: **Atlas of Pulmonary Pathology**

Kanel and Korula: **Atlas of Liver and Biliary Tract Pathology**

# ATLAS OF ORTHOPEDIC PATHOLOGY

**Lester E. Wold, M.D.**
Consultant in Pathology
Mayo Clinic
Rochester, Minnesota

**Richard A. McLeod, M.D.**
Consultant in Diagnostic Radiology
Mayo Clinic
Rochester, Minnesota

**Franklin H. Sim, M.D.**
Consultant in Orthopedic Surgery
Mayo Clinic
Rochester, Minnesota

**K. Krishnan Unni, M.B.B.S**
Consultant in Pathology
Mayo Clinic
Rochester, Minnesota

**W.B. SAUNDERS COMPANY**
*A Division of Harcourt Brace & Company*
Philadelphia ■ London ■ Toronto ■ Montreal ■ Sydney ■ Tokyo

**W.B. SAUNDERS COMPANY**
*A Division of*
*Harcourt Brace & Company*

The Curtis Center
Independence Square West
Philadelphia, Pennsylvania 19106

**Library of Congress Cataloging-in-Publication Data**

Atlas of orthopedic pathology / Lester E. Wold . . . [et al.].

p.      cm.

1. Bones—Diseases—Atlases.      2. Orthopedics—Atlases.
   I. Wold, Lester E. (Lester Eugene), 1949–
   [DNLM: 1. Bone Disease—pathology—atlases.
   WE 17 A880632]

RC930.A85 1990          616.7'107'0222—dc20          DNLM/DLC
ISBN 0–7216–2911–3                                              90–8129
                                                                            CIP

Editor:   Richard Zorab
Designer:   Joan Wendt
Production Manager:   Carolyn Naylor
Manuscript Editor:   Tom Gibbons
Illustration Coordinator:   Brett MacNaughton
Page Layout Artist:   Joan Wendt
Indexer:   Susan Thomas

ATLAS OF ORTHOPEDIC PATHOLOGY                    ISBN 0-7216-2911-3

Printed in the United States of America

Last digit is the print number:  9 8 7 6 5 4 3

*To*
*Patty, Paul and Barbara;*
*Chandra Shiela, Akhil,*
*Adit and Adosh; and Jan.*

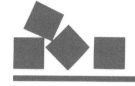

# PREFACE

This atlas of orthopedic tumors and tumor-like conditions is intended as an introduction to this complex subject. It offers a starting point for pathology residents, orthopedic residents, and radiology residents to learn about the clinical and pathologic features commonly encountered in patients with these conditions. The atlas is organized by condition into chapters, e.g., osteosarcoma, chondrosarcoma, etc. Each chapter is organized in the same way with information on the peak age, male-to-female ratio, and most common locations preceding a skeletal distribution and age diagram. Numbers on the skeletal distribution diagrams indicate the percentage of total cases occurring in that bone.

Clinical symptoms, clinical signs, major radiographic features, radiographic differential diagnosis, gross and microscopic pathologic features, pathologic differential diagnosis, and treatment sections are organized in each chapter in an outline format. Only the major features are presented. For more information the reader is referred to an abbreviated list of references that follows the outlined information. These references are by no means complete but, again, offer a starting point for a more in-depth review of any one of the conditions. Attempts have been made to include both older, key references and more recent reviews that encompass the majority of the important reports of each condition. This atlas complements many texts that contain abundant information concerning both tumors and tumor-like conditions.

Lester E. Wold
Richard A. McLeod
Franklin H. Sim
K. Krishnan Unni

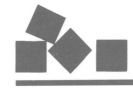

# ACKNOWLEDGMENTS

The authors gratefully acknowledge Drs. David C. Dahlin, John W. Beabout, and John C. Ivins, without whose helpful encouragement, counsel, and tutelage this book would not have been possible.

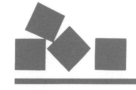

# CONTENTS

# Section 2

# Section 3

# SECTION ■ 1

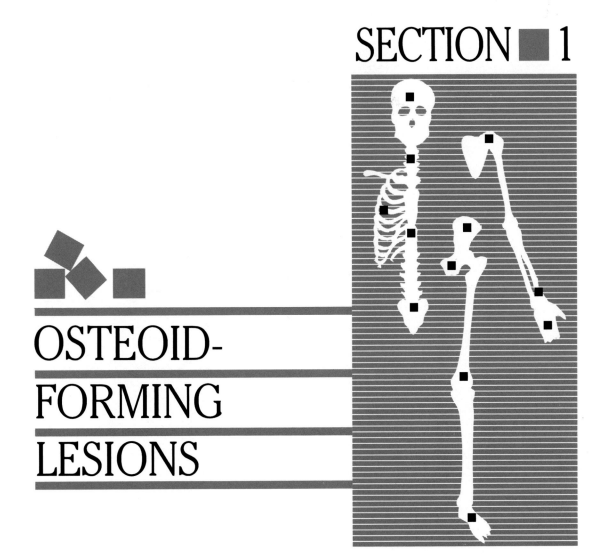

## OSTEOID-
## FORMING
## LESIONS

# CHAPTER 1

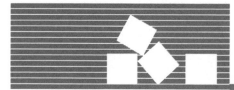

# Osteoid Osteoma

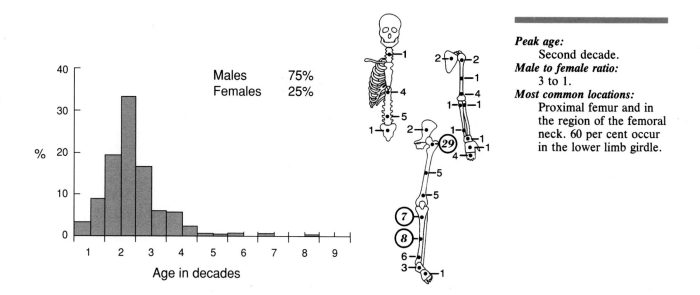

Males     75%
Females   25%

%    (vertical axis: 40, 30, 20, 10, 0)

Age in decades (horizontal axis: 1 2 3 4 5 6 7 8 9)

**Peak age:**
  Second decade.
**Male to female ratio:**
  3 to 1.
**Most common locations:**
  Proximal femur and in
  the region of the femoral
  neck. 60 per cent occur
  in the lower limb girdle.

## ■ Clinical Symptoms

1. The patient's complaints can be virtually diagnostic. The most important complaint is pain of increasing severity. The pain is frequently noted to be worse at night and is relieved with aspirin.
2. The pain may be referred to an adjacent joint.
3. If the involved bone is superficial, a painful local swelling may be noted.
4. If the tumor involves the vertebra, the patient may present with scoliosis.
5. Arthritic symptoms may be produced by tumors near a joint.

## ■ Clinical Signs

1. Lower extremity lesions will often cause dysfunction manifested as a limp.
2. Muscle atrophy may be present in the affected extremity.

3. Neurologic disorder may be suspected in some cases owing to the combination of pain, decreased muscle stretch reflexes, and muscular atrophy.
    Approximately 3 per cent of patients will have symptoms clinically suggestive of lumbar disc disease.

## ■ Major Radiographic Features

1. A small round lucency is identified on plane x-ray, usually lying in the cortex.
2. Surrounding the lucency are sclerosis and cortical reaction.
3. At the center of the lucency or nidus, there may be central ossification.
4. Twenty-five per cent of tumors are not demonstrated on plain x-ray and therefore require isotope bone scan, tomography, or computed tomography (CT) for identification.

5. Tumors in cancellous bone, subperiosteal tumors, and intracapsular tumors provoke little or no sclerosis.

■ **Radiographic Differential Diagnosis**

1. Brodie's abscess.
2. Stress fracture.
3. Osteoblastoma.

■ **Pathologic Features**

*Gross*

1. Lesional tissue is red in color.
2. The tumor is granular in texture but may be soft or densely sclerotic.
3. The nidus is generally very distinct from the surrounding sclerotic bone.
4. The lesional tissue is generally less than 1 cm in its greatest dimension.
5. The nidus may be difficult to identify grossly. In such cases tetracycline labeling preoperatively may be of help, since the nidus tends to stand out when viewed under ultraviolet light.

*Microscopic*

1. At low magnification the nidus consists of an interlacing network of osteoid trabeculae.
2. The trabeculae are usually thin and arranged in a haphazard manner.
3. Mineralization of the osteoid is variable, but the greatest degree of mineralization generally occurs at the center of the nidus.
4. Between the osteoid trabeculae there is a loose fibrovascular connective tissue.
5. Multinucleated giant cells may be identified within the fibrovascular connective tissue.
6. At higher magnification, the osteoblasts surrounding the osteoid trabeculae are uniform in their cytologic characteristics, having round regular nuclei and abundant cytoplasm.
7. Cartilage is not present.
8. The nidus is well demarcated from the surrounding bone, which generally has undergone sclerotic changes.

■ **Pathologic Differential Diagnosis**

Benign lesions:
1. Osteoblastoma.
Malignant lesions:
1. Osteosarcoma.

■ **Treatment**

**Primary Modality:** complete resection of the nidus with bone grafting as indicated, depending upon the size of the defect.

**Other Possible Considerations:** curettage, but this is to be discouraged because of the risk of leaving the nidus behind, leading to recurrence. Identification of the nidus may be facilitated by intraoperative bone scanning. Tetracycline labeling with ultraviolet light is useful for pathologic identification of the nidus.

**References**

McLeod RA, Dahlin DC, and Beabout, JW: The spectrum of osteoblastoma. Am J Roentgenol *126*:321–335, 1976.

Sim FH, Dahlin DC, and Beabout JW: Osteoid-osteoma: diagnostic problems. J Bone Joint Surg *57A*:154–159, 1975.

Sim FH, Dahlin DC, Stauffer RN, and Laws ER Jr: Primary bone tumors simulating lumbar disc syndrome. Spine *2*:65–74, 1977.

Swee RG, McLeod RA, and Beabout JW: Osteoid osteoma: detection, diagnosis and localization. Radiology *130*:117–123, 1979.

Vigorita VJ, and Ghelman B: Localization of osteoid osteomas—use of radionuclide scanning and autoimaging in identifying the nidus. Am J Clin Pathol *79*:223–225, 1983.

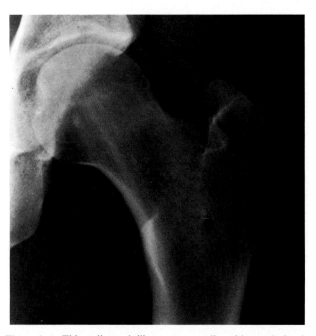

**Figure 1–1.** This radiograph illustrates a small oval lucent lesion in the intertrochanteric region of the femur. The radiographic features are compatible with the diagnosis of osteoid osteoma.

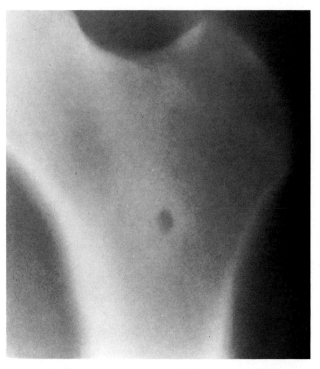

**Figure 1–2.** Tomograms may be helpful in evaluating such lesions. The surrounding sclerosis is identifiable.

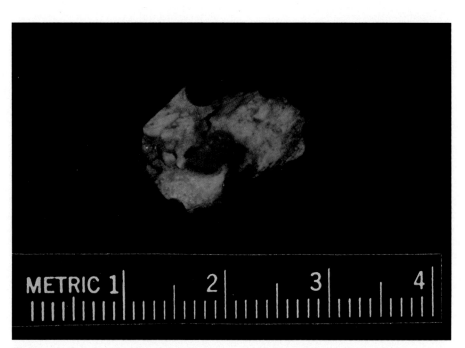

**Figure 1–3.** Grossly the nidus of osteoid osteoma is reddish and appears hemorrhagic, as shown in this photograph. The nidus tends to stand out from the surrounding sclerotic bone.

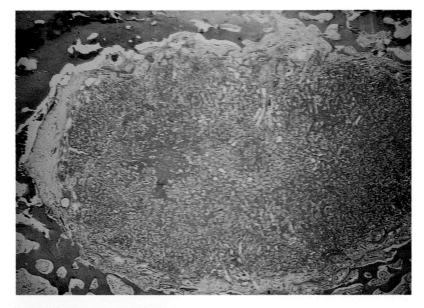

**Figure 1–4.** At low magnification the nidus of osteoid osteoma is well circumscribed. The surrounding bone is sclerotic, a reactive change that may extend for a considerable distance from the nidus.

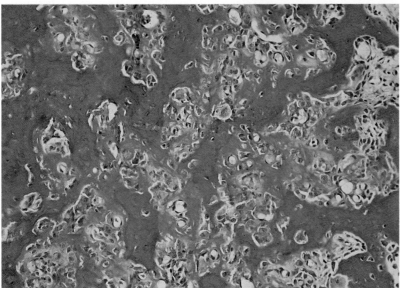

**Figure 1–5.** At the center of the nidus the lesion is composed of irregular trabeculae of bone, which lie in a hypocellular, fibrovascular connective tissue. These features are identical with those of osteoblastoma.

**Figure 1–6.** At high magnification the irregularity of the osteoid and the cellular proliferation may be misinterpreted as representing an osteosarcoma. Using low power and paying attention to the radiographic features help the pathologist avoid this mistake.

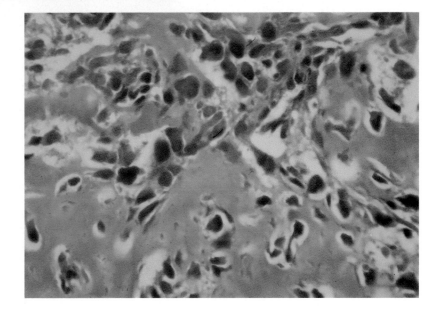

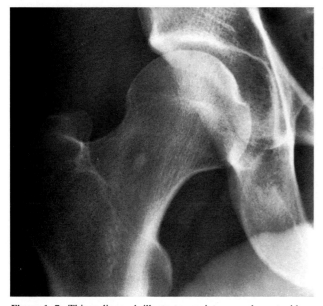

**Figure 1-7.** This radiograph illustrates an intracapsular osteoid osteoma of the femoral neck. The central ossification is typical of this lesion; however, the tumor has not provoked any surrounding sclerosis.

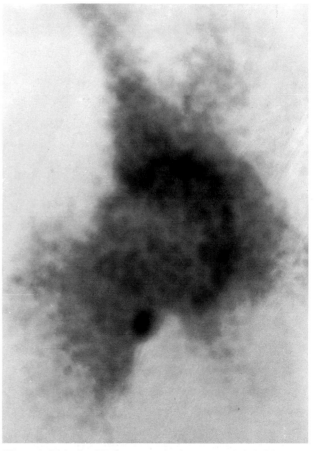

**Figure 1-9.** An isotope bone scan is also extremely helpful in identifying small osteoid osteomas that are radiographically inapparent, as this bone scan illustrates.

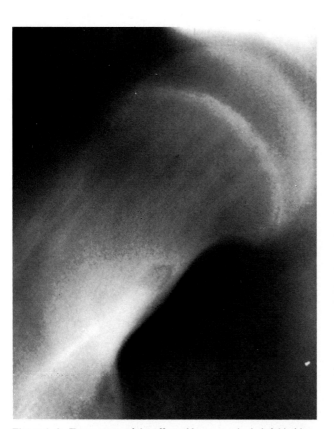

**Figure 1-8.** Tomograms of the affected bone may be helpful in identifying the nidus in cases where the plain x-ray is unrevealing. Sclerosis surrounds the nidus seen in this tomogram of the proximal femur.

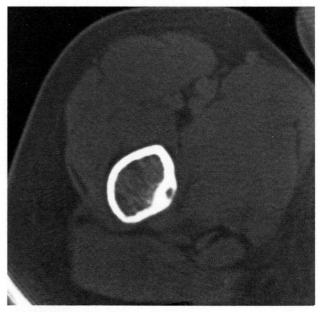

**Figure 1-10.** A CT scan may also be helpful in some cases. In this case a cortical subtrochanteric osteoid osteoma of the femur was identified using a CT scan.

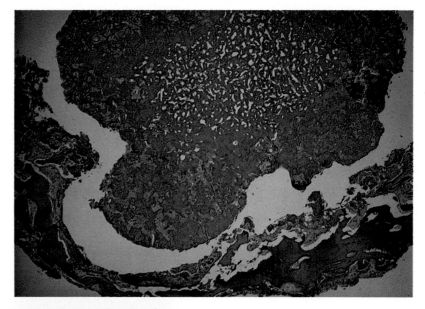

**Figure 1–11.** Some osteoid osteomas show extensive ossification of the nidus, as illustrated in this photomicrograph. Note the marked circumscription, which results in the lesion appearing to "break away" from the surrounding bone.

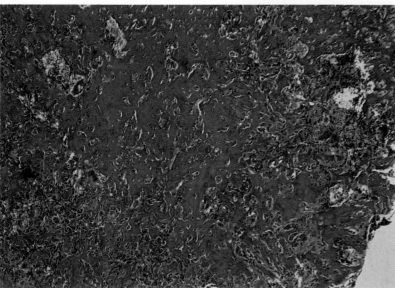

**Figure 1–12.** In cases with extensive ossification of the nidus, cytologic evaluation of the lesion is difficult.

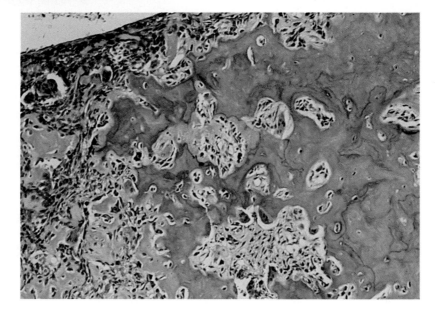

**Figure 1–13.** At higher magnification the histologic features may resemble those of pagetoid bone. Attention to the radiographic features helps to avoid a misdiagnosis in such cases.

# CHAPTER 2

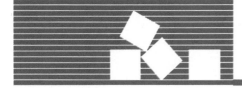

# Osteoblastoma

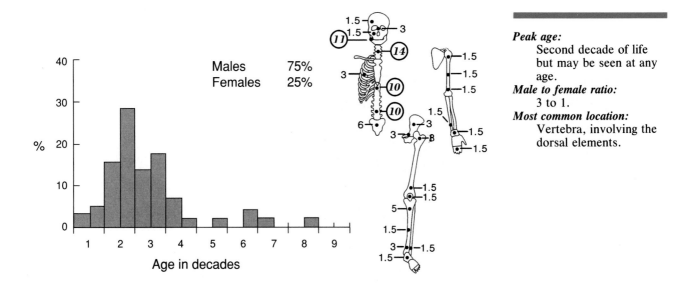

Males 75%
Females 25%

% — Age in decades

*Peak age:*
Second decade of life but may be seen at any age.
*Male to female ratio:*
3 to 1.
*Most common location:*
Vertebra, involving the dorsal elements.

■ **Clinical Symptoms**

1. Local pain is generally the presenting complaint and is usually of long duration.
2. The pain may follow the characteristic pattern of osteoid osteoma, but more commonly does not.
3. Patients with lesions in the lower extremity may present with a limp.
4. Rarely patients have presented with severe systemic symptoms, which were ameliorated by radical treatment of the tumor.

■ **Clinical Signs**

1. A tender mass lesion may be found on physical examination.
2. Scoliosis or atrophy of muscle groups in the region of the tumor may be present.
3. Neurologic deficit may be appreciable owing to vertebral tumors compressing the cord or nerve roots.

■ **Major Radiographic Features**

1. The radiographic features may be similar to those of osteoid osteoma.
2. The appearance is quite variable and may be non-specific.
3. Twenty-five per cent of cases show features suggestive of a malignant neoplasm.
4. In the vertebra, osteoblastoma usually results in expansion and is located in the dorsal elements. Fifty per cent show ossification radiographically.
5. Mandibular lesions (cementoblastoma) are "ossified," surrounded by a lucent halo, and located near a tooth root.

■ **Radiographic Differential Diagnosis**

1. Osteoid osteoma.
2. Osteosarcoma.
3. Aneurysmal bone cyst.

## ■ Pathologic Features

### Gross

1. The lesional tissue is hemorrhagic and reddish in color.
2. The tissue is granular and friable in quality.
3. At its periphery the tumor shows sharp circumscription.
4. The tumor may bleed profusely when curetted owing to its extensive vasculature.

### Microscopic

1. At low magnification the pattern of the tumor is that of irregular osteoid arranged haphazardly amid a loose fibrovascular connective tissue.
2. The vascular component is obvious at low magnification with wide lumina.
3. Prominent osteoblastic rimming of the osteoid is evident.
4. The periphery of the lesion is well circumscribed, but the osteoid may merge with the adjacent normal bone.
5. At higher magnification, the osteoblasts are uniform but do not totally fill the intertrabecular space.
6. The osteoid may be quite fine and "lace-like" as is seen in osteosarcoma, but cartilaginous differentiation is not present.
7. Mitotic figures may be identified and may be quite numerous, but atypical mitoses are not present.

## ■ Pathologic Differential Diagnosis

Benign lesions:
1. Osteoid osteoma.
2. Aneurysmal bone cyst.
Malignant lesions:
1. Osteosarcoma.

## ■ Treatment

**Primary Modality:** curettage and grafting.
**Other Possible Approaches:** en bloc resection with a marginal margin and grafting, depending on location. Spinal lesions may require complete removal by excision or curettage, preserving nerve roots. Bone grafting to stabilize the vertebral column is often necessary.

## References

Bertoni F, Unni KK, McLeod RA, and Dahlin DC: Osteosarcoma resembling osteoblastoma. Cancer 55:416–426, 1985.

Dorfman JD, and Weiss SW: Borderline osteoblastic tumors: problems in the differential diagnosis of aggressive osteoblastoma and low-grade osteosarcoma. Semin Diagn Pathol 1:215–234, 1984.

Jackson RP, Reckling FW, and Mants FA: Osteoid osteoma and osteoblastoma: similar histologic lesions with different natural histories. Clin Orthop 128:303–313, 1977.

McLeod RA, Dahlin DC, and Beabout JW: The spectrum of osteoblastoma. Am J Roentgenol 126:321–335, 1976.

Mirra JM, Kendrick RA, and Kendrick RE: Pseudomalignant osteoblastoma versus arrested osteosarcoma: a case report. Cancer 37:2005–2014, 1976.

Mirra JM, Theros E, Smasson J, et al: A case of osteoblastoma associated with severe systemic toxicity. Am J Surg Pathol 3:463–471, 1979.

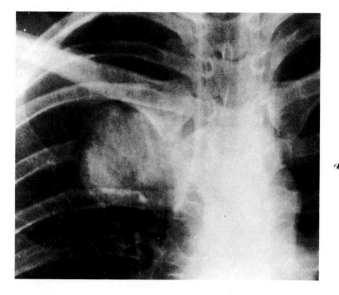

**Figure 2–1.** This radiograph illustrates a partially ossified mass lesion involving a rib posteriorly. There is associated bone destruction and a soft tissue mass indicative of an aggressive lesion.

**Figure 2–2.** The CT scan in this case illustrates the same features that are evident in the plain x-ray.

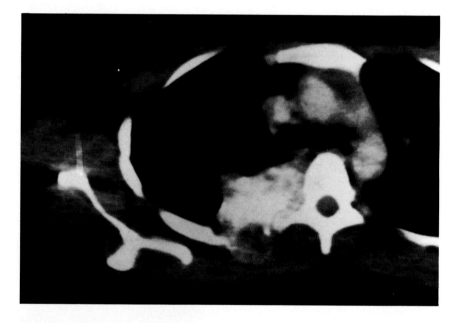

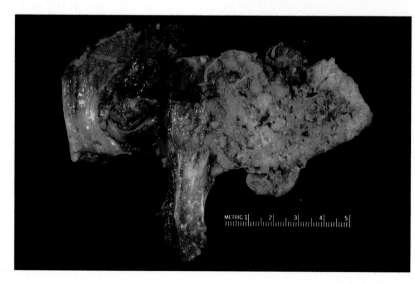

**Figure 2–3.** The gross pathologic features in this case correlate well with the plain x-ray and CT appearance of the lesion. The tumor was confirmed histologically to be an osteoblastoma.

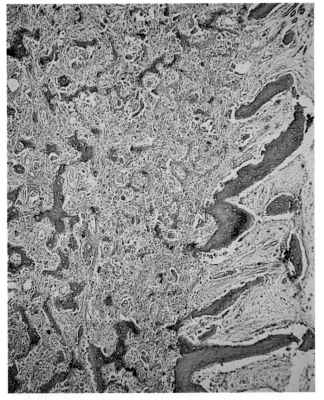

**Figure 2–4.** At low magnification the periphery of an osteoblastoma is well circumscribed, as is illustrated in this photomicrograph.

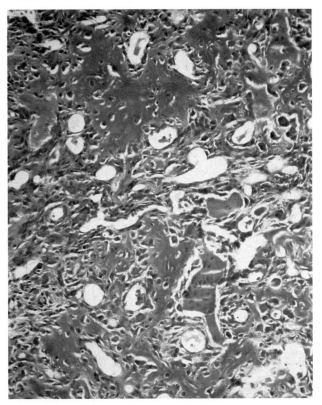

**Figure 2–6.** Numerous multinucleated giant cells and a prominent osteoblastic rimming of the bony trabeculae are evident. Vascular spaces are generally prominent.

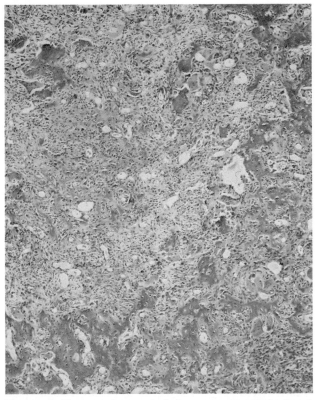

**Figure 2–5.** The tumor is composed of numerous irregularly shaped bony trabeculae between which there is hypocellular fibrovascular connective tissue.

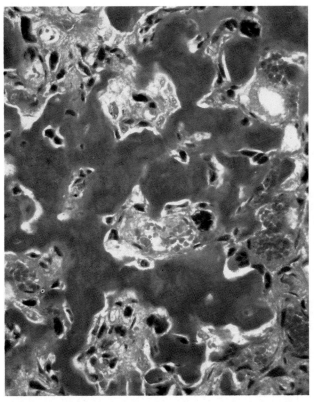

**Figure 2–7.** At high magnification, the lesion is not hypercellular and nuclear pleomorphism is generally not marked. However, some lesions can show cytologic changes that may simulate osteosarcoma, as is illustrated in this photomicrograph.

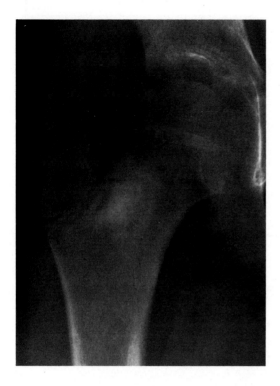

**Figure 2–8.** This radiograph of the proximal femur illustrates the appearance of a heavily ossified oval osteoblastoma. A lucent halo surrounds the ossified lesion and is itself surrounded by a zone of sclerosis—features that support a benign diagnosis.

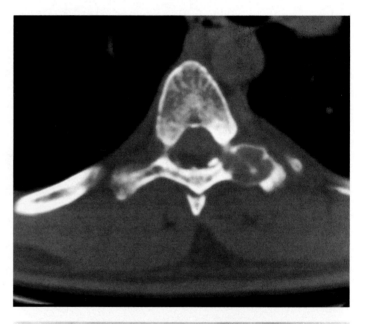

**Figure 2–9.** Osteoblastomas commonly involve the vertebrae; the dorsal elements are usually the location of such lesions, as is illustrated in this case. The central ossification is also characteristic of this tumor.

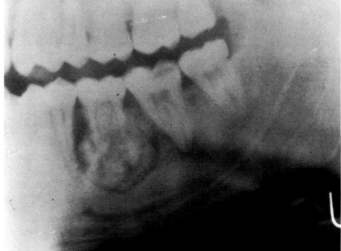

**Figure 2–10.** Lesions histologically indistinguishable from osteoblastoma also involve the maxilla and mandible, as illustrated in this case. Such lesions have been termed "cementoblastomas." Note the ossified tumor surrounding the tooth root with a lucent halo.

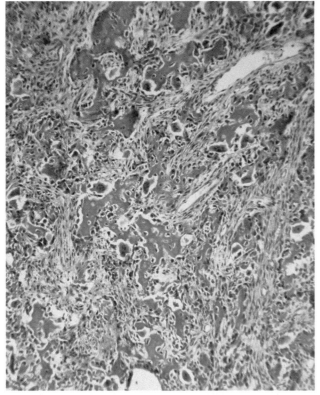

**Figure 2–11.** Although the irregular bony trabeculae of osteoblastoma may simulate the osteoid produced by osteosarcomas, the hypocellular nature of the fibrovascular connective tissue seen between such trabeculae supports a diagnosis of osteoblastoma.

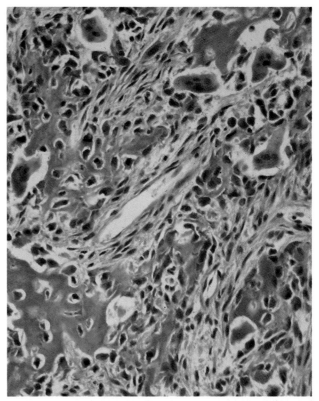

**Figure 2–13.** Careful attention should be paid to the appearance of the lesion at low magnification and to the radiographic features, as overemphasis of the high-power appearance of a lesion may lead to a mistaken diagnosis of malignancy.

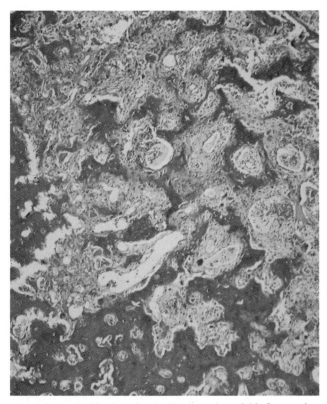

**Figure 2–12.** Ossification of osteoblastomas is variable from region to region in the tumor. This photomicrograph illustrates the transition from a more heavily ossified area to a less ossified region.

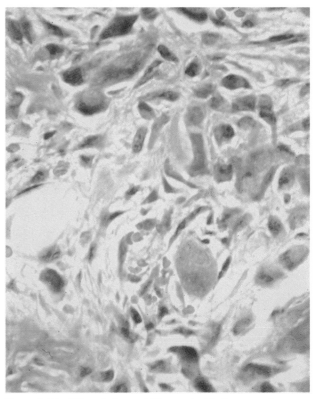

**Figure 2–14.** Although the nuclei in an osteoblastoma may be somewhat hyperchromatic, the cells do not lie "shoulder-to-shoulder" as in an osteosarcoma. Thus the osteoblastoma has a looser appearance, as is illustrated in this photomicrograph.

# CHAPTER 3

## Osteosarcoma (Conventional)

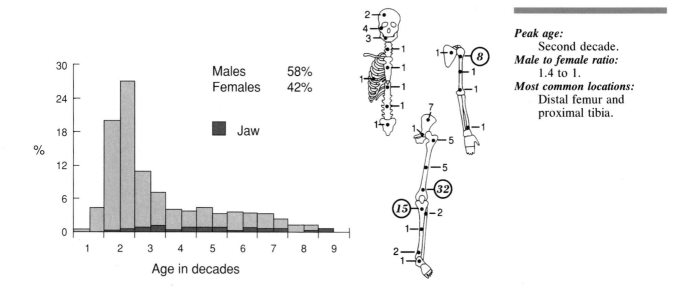

Males 58%
Females 42%

■ Jaw

% 

Age in decades

*Peak age:*
  Second decade.
*Male to female ratio:*
  1.4 to 1.
*Most common locations:*
  Distal femur and
  proximal tibia.

■ **Clinical Symptoms**

1. Pain, which may be intermittent initially, is universally present.
2. A swelling in the region of the affected bone is also a cardinal, although nonspecific, symptom.
3. Pathologic fracture is uncommon as the presenting complaint.
4. The duration of symptoms is generally short, varying from weeks to several months.

■ **Clinical Signs**

1. A tender mass generally is palpable on physical examination, since soft tissue extension is common.
2. When the mass is very large, dilated and engorged veins may be seen overlying it.
3. Edema distal to the lesion due to blockage of lymphatics or venous compression occurs uncommonly.
4. Elevation of serum alkaline phosphatase concentrations occurs in about 50 per cent of patients.

■ **Major Radiographic Features**

1. The favored site is the metaphysis of a long bone, especially the knee.
2. It may be lytic, blastic, or mixed bone destruction and production.
3. Trabecular and cortical destruction is usually geographic and poorly marginated.
4. Periosteal new bone is frequent and often takes the form of spiculation or Codman's triangles.
5. Soft tissue extension is the rule in larger lesions.
6. Magnetic resonance imaging (MRI) and computed tomography (CT) are essential for pretreatment staging.

### ■ Radiographic Differential Diagnosis

1. Ewing's sarcoma.
2. Fibrosarcoma/malignant fibrous histiocytoma.
3. Chondrosarcoma.
4. Osteomyelitis.
5. Osteoblastoma.
6. Giant cell tumor.

### ■ Pathologic Features

#### Gross

1. The tumors generally have violated the cortex of the affected bone at the time of diagnosis.
2. An associated soft tissue mass is commonly found.
3. The tumor may extend within the medullary cavity beyond the abnormality defined by plane x-ray (magnetic resonance imaging [MRI] is particularly helpful in defining the extent of intramedullary disease).
4. The tumor is variable in consistency and may be distinctly sclerotic; in general, however, soft areas are identifiable as well.
5. The tumor varies in color from yellow-brown to whitish, depending upon whether the predominant differentiation is fibroblastic, chondroblastic, or osteoblastic.
6. Necrosis, cyst formation, and hemorrhage are most commonly seen in the softer portions of the tumor.

#### Microscopic

1. At low magnification the tumor may show great variability. However, all tumors classified as osteosarcoma must show a frankly sarcomatous stroma that produces osteoid (frequently the osteoid shows a fine lace-like pattern).
2. The tumor is hypercellular, and generally the stromal cells are spindled in shape.
3. Zones of chrondroid matrix may be identified.
4. Sclerotic zones of extensive ossification may appear hypocellular, having undergone degeneration.
5. The spindle cells may be arranged in a "herring bone" or storiform pattern.
6. At higher magnification the spindled cells show marked pleomorphism. The nuclei are extremely variable in size and shape and are hyperchromic.
7. Mitotic figures are generally abundant.
8. The degree to which osteoid is produced is extremely variable, and a careful search may need to be made in order to identify the eosinophilic matrix surrounding atypical cells.
9. Variable numbers of benign multinucleated giant cells are seen; when abundant, they may focally mimic the appearance of a giant cell tumor.

### ■ Pathologic Differential Diagnosis

Benign lesions:
1. Osteoblastoma.
2. Osteoid osteoma.
3. Giant cell tumor.
4. Fracture callus.
Malignant lesions:
1. Fibrosarcoma.
2. Chondrosarcoma.
3. Malignant fibrous histiocytoma.

### ■ Treatment

**Primary Modality:** surgical ablation by amputation or limb-saving resection with a wide margin. If preoperative staging indicates that a successful limb-salvage procedure can be performed, the extremity can be reconstructed with a custom joint prosthesis, an osteochondral allograft, or a resection arthrodesis. The reconstructive procedure should be tailored to the needs of the individual. Clinical trials with various chemotherapeutic agents—usually including high-dose methotrexate, doxorubicin, or cis-platinum—are currently in progress. Protocols utilizing preoperative (neoadjuvant) chemotherapy use the extent of tumor "necrosis" at the time of definitive operation as a measure of effectiveness. Current advances in chemotherapy are making an important contribution to the improved survival of patients with osteosarcoma. An aggressive approach with thoracotomy is salvaging approximately one-third of the patients who develop pulmonary metastases.

**Other Possible Approaches:** radiation therapy, possibly combined with neutron beam radiation for lesions of inaccessible sites such as the spine and sacrum.

### References

Campanacci M, Bacci G, Bertoni F, et al: The treatment of osteosarcoma of the extremities: twenty years experience at the Istituto Ortopedico Rizzoli. Cancer 48:1569–1581, 1981.

Harvei S, and Solheim O: The prognosis in osteosarcoma: Norwegian national data. Cancer 48:1719–1723, 1981.

Marcove RC, and Rosen G: En bloc resection for osteogenic sarcoma. Cancer 45:3040–3044, 1980.

Martin SE, Dwyer A, Kissane JM, and Cost J: Small-cell osteosarcoma. Cancer 50:990–996, 1982.

Sanerkin NG: Definitions of osteosarcoma, chondrosarcoma and fibrosarcoma of bone. Cancer 46:178–185, 1980.

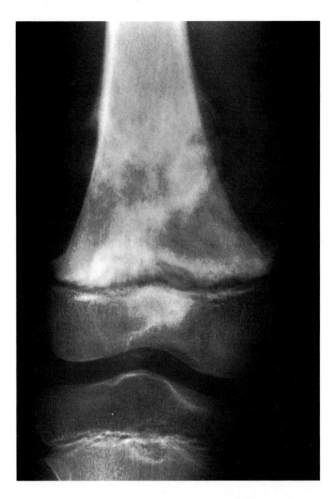

**Figure 3–1.** This anteroposterior radiograph demonstrates a mixed lytic and sclerotic lesion in the distal femur of a skeletally immature patient. Codman's triangle is present superiorly. The radiographic features are those of an osteosarcoma.

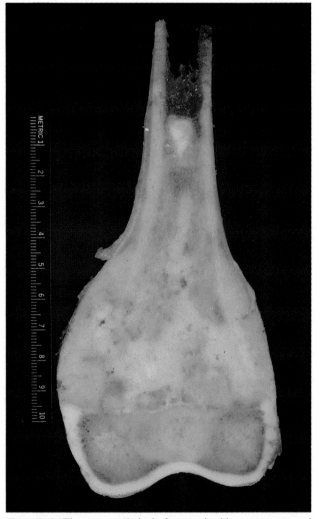

**Figure 3–2.** The gross pathologic features in this case correspond well with the plain x-ray appearance shown above. The tumor crosses the open physis, which often acts as a relative barrier to the intraosseous extension of osteosarcomas. The tumor is firm and gritty; however, soft areas are nearly always present.

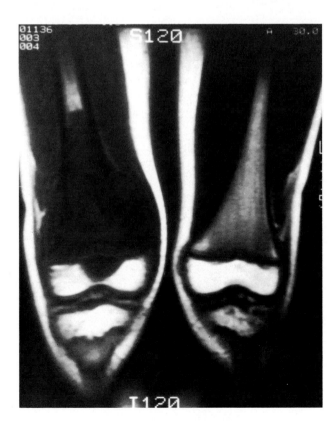

**Figure 3–3.** This coronal MRI of the same patient's distal femur demonstrates the extent of the low-signal tumor seen in contrast to the high-signal normal marrow. The extension of the tumor across the physis into the epiphysis is also readily demonstrated.

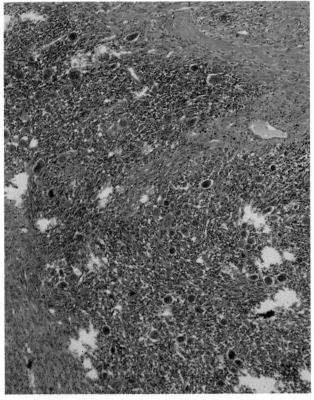

**Figure 3–4.** At low magnification osteosarcomas show a variety of histologic patterns. This photomicrograph illustrates a tumor that is predominantly composed of spindle cells (fibroblastic) in which numerous benign multinucleated giant cells are present.

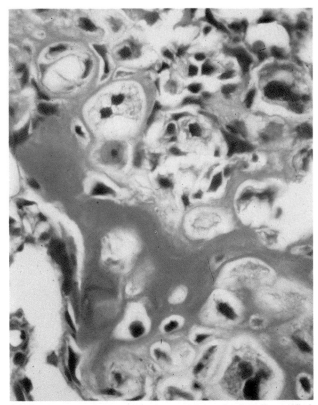

**Figure 3–6.** Osteoblastic osteosarcomas may be heavily ossified; however, the cytologic atypia of the proliferating cells is generally obvious in such cases, as is shown in this photomicrograph.

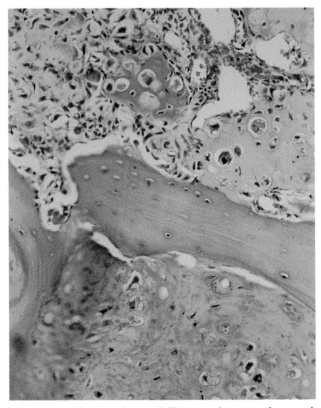

**Figure 3–5.** This photomicrograph illustrates the permeative growth of a chondroblastic osteosarcoma of the distal femur. Residual bony trabeculae are present. The chondroid portion of such a tumor may not show as significant cytologic atypia as the spindle cell components of the lesion and thus, if taken out of context, may suggest the diagnosis of chondrosarcoma.

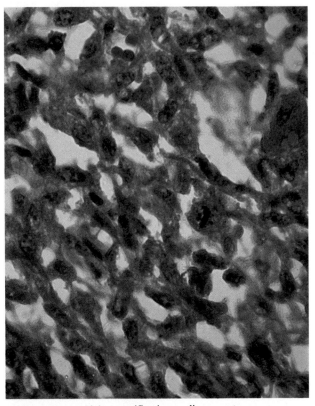

**Figure 3–7.** At high magnification ordinary osteosarcomas are poorly differentiated or high-grade tumors. They show nuclear pleomorphism and anaplasia, and mitotic activity is generally brisk.

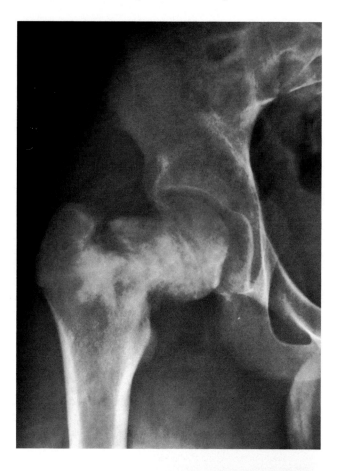

**Figure 3–8.** This radiograph of the proximal femur shows a sclerotic osteosarcoma that has resulted in a pathologic fracture.

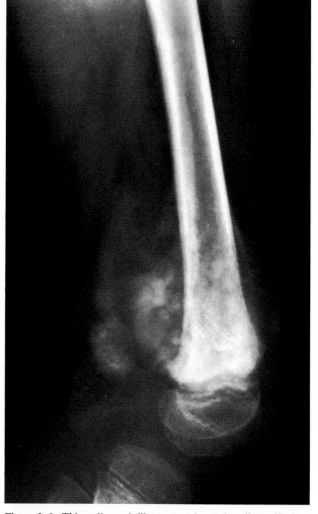

**Figure 3–9.** This radiograph illustrates a large, heavily ossified osteosarcoma of the lower femoral metaphysis with a large soft tissue component.

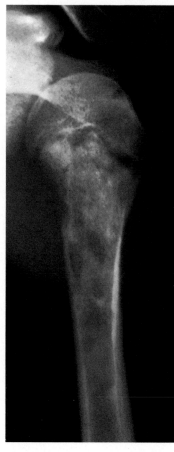

**Figure 3–10.** A mixed lytic and sclerotic radiographic appearance is common in osteosarcoma, as is illustrated in this case involving the upper diametaphyseal region of the humerus.

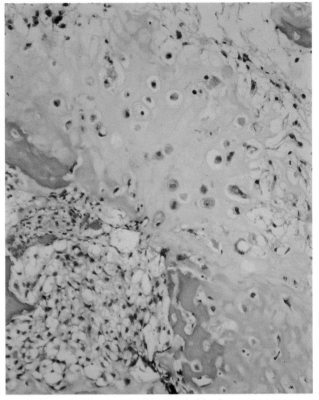

**Figure 3–11.** Ossification within a chondroblastic osteosarcoma may occur at the periphery of the cartilaginous masses, as is illustrated in this photomicrograph, or within a spindle cell component of the lesion.

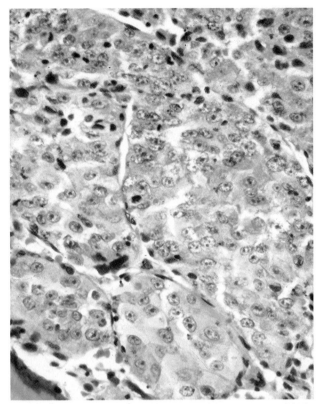

**Figure 3–13.** Some osteosarcomas show a distinctly epithelioid histologic pattern of growth, as is illustrated in this photomicrograph of a tumor from the radius. Given the young age of most patients with osteosarcoma, such a pattern generally does not result in misdiagnosis.

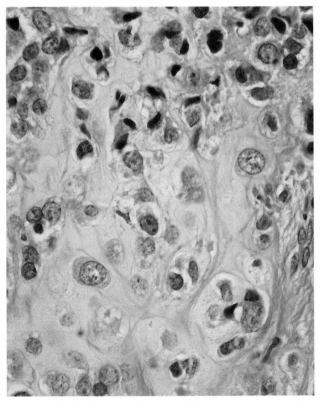

**Figure 3–12.** At high magnification ordinary osteosarcomas show marked cytologic atypia. The "lace-like" osteoid that identifies the tumor as an osteosarcoma may be only focally present.

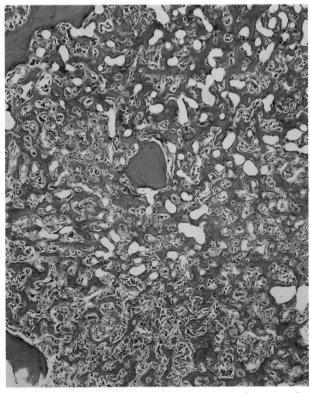

**Figure 3–14.** Postchemotherapy osteosarcomas may show extensive regions of ossification, without identifiable viable tumor. The soft tissue and peripheral components of the tumor are the areas in which viable tumor is most commonly identified after chemotherapy.

# CHAPTER 4

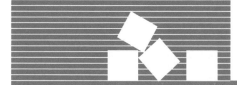

# Parosteal Osteosarcoma

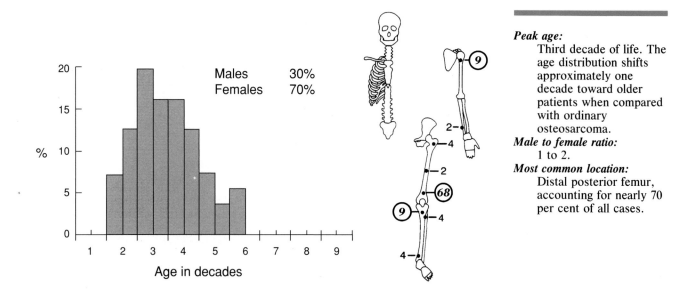

Males 30%
Females 70%

% 

Age in decades

**Peak age:**
Third decade of life. The age distribution shifts approximately one decade toward older patients when compared with ordinary osteosarcoma.

**Male to female ratio:**
1 to 2.

**Most common location:**
Distal posterior femur, accounting for nearly 70 per cent of all cases.

■ **Clinical Symptoms**

1. A painless mass is present in the posterior distal thigh.
2. The mass is generally of long duration (up to several years).
3. Some patients complain of inability to bend the knee if the mass is sufficiently large.
4. Pain is uncommon.

■ **Major Radiographic Features**

1. A lobulated and ossified mass arises on the metaphyseal surface of a long bone.
2. The posterior lower femur is a preferred site.
3. There is broad attachment to the adjacent cortex.
4. The cortex is thickened and deformed.
5. Larger tumors encircle the bone.

■ **Radiographic Differential Diagnosis**

1. Myositis ossificans
2. Periosteal osteosarcoma.
3. Periosteal chondrosarcoma.
4. High-grade surface osteosarcoma.
5. Ordinary osteosarcoma.
6. Osteochondroma.

■ **Clinical Signs**

1. A large mass lesion involves the affected bone.
2. The tumor may be tender to palpation.

■ **Pathologic Features**

*Gross*

1. The tumor seems to be applied to the surface of the affected bone.
2. Medullary extension is absent unless the tumor

is recurrent or has been present for many years.
3. The tumor is ossified and rock-hard; if soft areas exist, they should be sampled since the tumor may have a higher-grade component in it.
4. Cartilaginous foci may be grossly evident and may form a "cap" over the tumor similar to an osteochondroma.

### Microscopic

1. At low magnification the pattern is that of a low-grade tumor. Osteoid trabeculae lie parallel to one another in a hypocellular, fibroblastic stroma.
2. The fibroblastic component of the tumor shows minimal cytologic atypia, and only rare mitoses are present.
3. At the surface of the tumor a cartilaginous cap may be present, giving the tumor the appearance of an osteochondroma. However, between the bony trabeculae of an osteochondroma there is fatty or hematopoietic marrow, in contrast with the fibrous stroma of a parosteal osteosarcoma. In addition, the chondrocytes show mild cytologic atypia and do not exhibit the columnar arrangement seen in an osteochondroma.

### ■ Pathologic Differential Diagnosis

Benign lesions:
1. Osteochondroma.
2. Myositis ossificans (heterotopic ossification).

Malignant lesions:
1. High-grade surface osteosarcoma.
2. Periosteal osteosarcoma.

### ■ Treatment

**Primary Modality:** limb-saving resection with a wide surgical margin and skeletal reconstruction with a custom prosthesis, osteochondral allograft, or resection arthrodesis.

**Other Possible Approaches:** amputation if an adequate margin cannot be achieved by resection owing to size or neurovascular involvement. Chemotherapy is probably not indicated in this variant of osteosarcoma.

### References

Ahuja SC, Villacin AB, Smith J, et al: Juxtacortical (parosteal) osteogenic sarcoma: histological grading and prognosis. J Bone Joint Surg 59A:632–647, 1977.

Edeiken J, Farrell C, Ackerman LV, and Spjut HJ: Parosteal sarcoma. Am J Roentgenol 111:579–583, 1971.

Unni KK, Dahlin DC, and Beabout JW: Periosteal osteogenic sarcoma. Cancer 37:2476–2485, 1976.

Unni KK, Dahlin DC, Beabout JW, and Ivins JC: Parosteal osteogenic sarcoma. Cancer 37:2466–2475, 1976.

Wold LE, Unni KK, Beabout JW, et al: Dedifferentiated parosteal osteosarcoma. J Bone Joint Surg 66A:53–59, 1984.

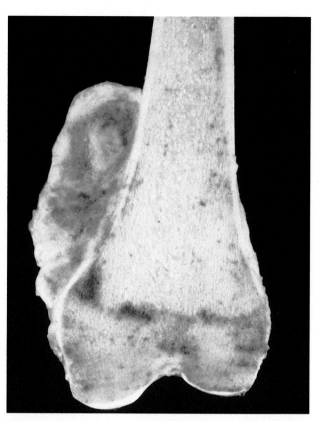

**Figure 4–2.** The gross pathologic features of this resected specimen correlate well with its radiographic appearance (see Fig. 4–1). The tumor is densely ossified and no medullary involvement is present. Any soft areas of the tumor should be sampled as they may represent ''transformation'' of the tumor.

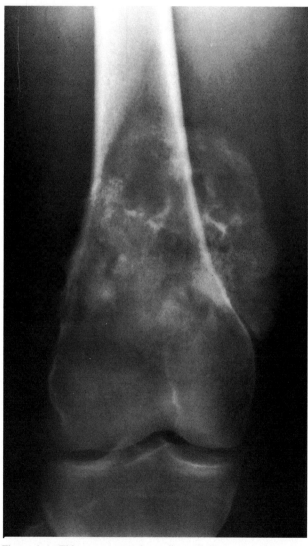

**Figure 4–1.** This anteroposterior radiograph illustrates the typical features of a parosteal osteosarcoma. The tumor is heavily ossified and broadly attached to the surface of the bone.

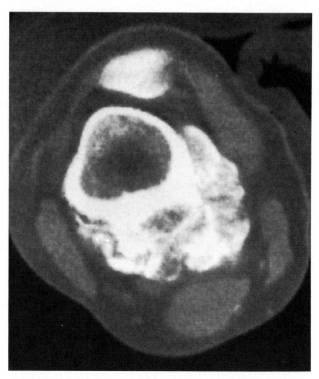

**Figure 4–3.** A CT scan of the tumor may be helpful in excluding medullary involvement. This scan shows the broad surface attachment of a parosteal osteosarcoma and the absence of medullary neoplasm.

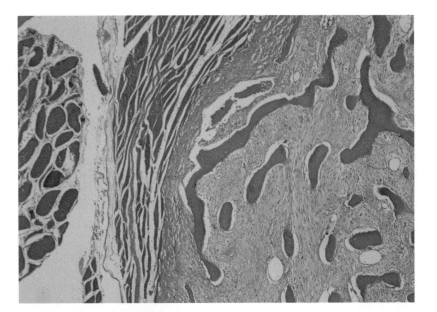

**Figure 4–4.** At low magnification parosteal osteosarcoma shows an orderly appearance, with a hypocellular spindle cell component merging with mature-appearing, "normalized" bony trabeculae. The periphery of the lesion is generally well circumscribed, as shown in this photomicrograph.

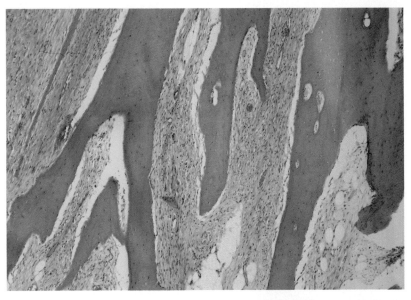

**Figure 4–5.** At higher magnification the cytologic features of the spindle cell component of the tumor are more apparent. The juxtaposition of hypocellular spindle cells and mature bone may simulate the histologic features of fibrous dysplasia.

**Figure 4–6.** At high magnification minimal cytologic atypia is apparent in the spindle cell component of the tumor.

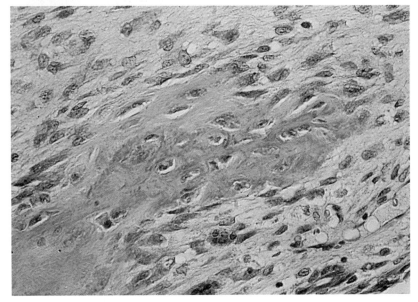

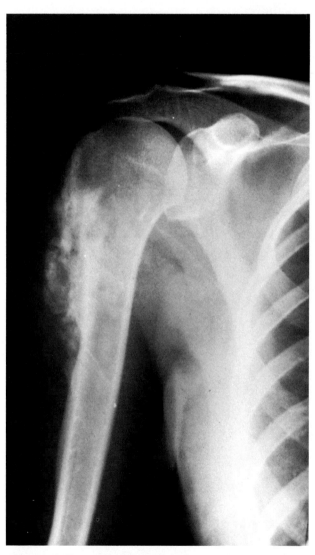

**Figure 4–7.** The proximal humerus is the second most common location for parosteal osteosarcoma. This tumor shows the characteristic broad-based bony attachment.

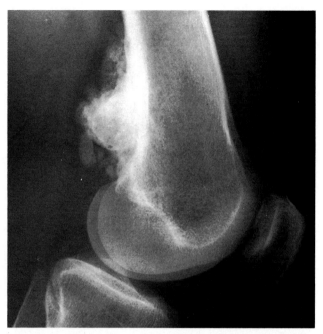

**Figure 4–8.** The distal posterior femur is the most common location for parosteal osteosarcoma. Medullary involvement is not identified in this lateral radiograph.

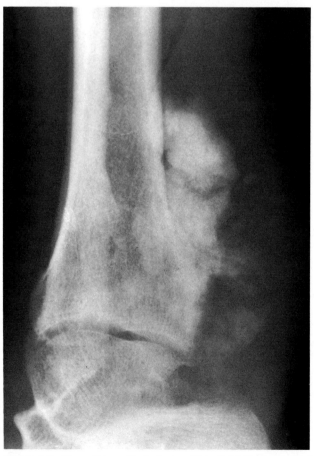

**Figure 4–9.** The radiographic features of this distal tibial parosteal osteosarcoma are identical with those of tumors in the more common locations.

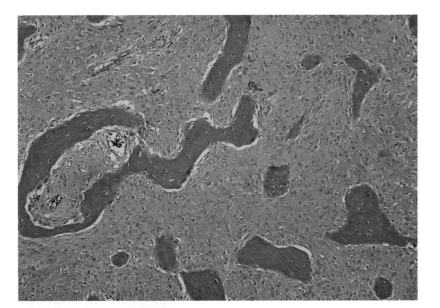

**Figure 4–10.** Irregular "matured" bony trabeculae of parosteal osteosarcoma may simulate the low-power pattern of fibrous dysplasia. However, the surface location of the lesion excludes the diagnosis of fibrous dysplasia.

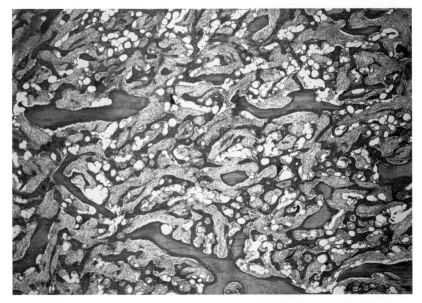

**Figure 4–11.** In recurrent or long-standing cases of parosteal osteosarcoma the medullary cavity may be involved, as is shown in this case. The well differentiated neoplasm is identified permeating the pre-existing medullary bony trabeculae.

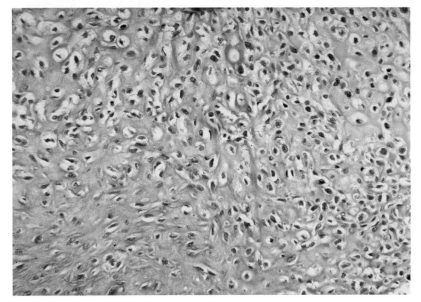

**Figure 4–12.** Any soft areas in a lesion that otherwise has the features of parosteal osteosarcoma should be histologically examined. This photomicrograph illustrates such a region in a recurrent tumor. The spindle cell proliferation shows much greater cytologic atypia than is seen in parosteal osteosarcoma. Such tumors have been termed "dedifferentiated parosteal osteosarcoma."

# CHAPTER 5

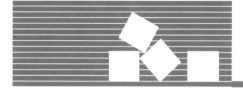

# Periosteal Osteosarcoma

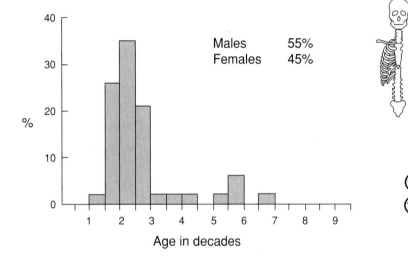

Males    55%
Females  45%

% / Age in decades

*Peak age:*
  Second decade.
*Male to female ratio:*
  Slight female
  predominance.
*Most common location:*
  Diaphysis of the femur
  and tibia.

■ **Clinical Symptoms**

1. Pain is the most common presenting complaint.
2. A swelling may be noticed by the patient.

■ **Clinical Signs**

1. A mass may be palpable on physical examination.
2. The lesion may be tender to palpation.

■ **Major Radiographic Features**

1. The lesion is diaphyseal in location, particularly in the tibia.
2. It is located on the surface of the bone; the medullary canal is uninvolved.
3. Partial matrix mineralization may be seen.
4. The periphery of the soft tissue mass is free of mineral.
5. The adjacent cortex is thickened.

6. Periosteal reaction and Codman's triangle are common.

■ **Radiographic Differential Diagnosis**

1. Parosteal osteosarcoma.
2. High-grade surface osteosarcoma.
3. Periosteal chondrosarcoma.
4. Myositis ossificans (heterotopic ossification).

■ **Pathologic Features**

*Gross*

1. The tumor is lobulated, situated on the surface of the bone, and may appear like a piece of putty applied to the periosteum.
2. The blue-gray color of a hyaline cartilage tumor is apparent.
3. Whitish spicules of bone may be seen to radiate through the tumor at right angles to the long axis of the underlying bone.
4. The medullary cavity is uninvolved.

*Microscopic*

1. At low magnification the tumor shows abundant chondroid matrix production.
2. Traversing the chondroid matrix are spicules of osteoid.
3. The periphery is generally well circumscribed, and the tumor shows lobulation in these regions.
4. At the periphery of the lesion the tumor shows a "condensation" of spindle-shaped cells.
5. At higher magnification the cells lying within the chondroid matrix show mild cytologic atypia.
6. The spindled cells at the periphery also show cytologic atypia, and faint osteoid may be seen among them.
7. The cortical bone may be slightly eroded, but the medullary canal is free of tumor.
8. Mitotic activity is not brisk.

## ■ Pathologic Differential Diagnosis

Benign lesions:
1. Periosteal chondroma.
Malignant lesions:
1. Periosteal chondrosarcoma.
2. High-grade surface osteosarcoma.
3. Ordinary intramedullary osteosarcoma with a prominent surface component.

## ■ Treatment

**Primary Modality:** This lesion lends itself to surgical resection with a wide margin, and the bone can be reconstructed utilizing an intercalary allograft or a vascularized fibular graft.

**Other Possible Approaches:** When an adequate margin cannot be achieved by en bloc resection, amputation is indicated. Preoperative chemotherapy may improve the low risk for local recurrence after local resection.

## References

Bertoni F, Boriani S, Laus M, and Campanacci M: Periosteal chondrosarcoma and periosteal osteosarcoma: two distinct entities. J Bone Joint Surg *64B*:370–376, 1982.

Unni KK, Dahlin DC, and Beabout JW: Periosteal osteogenic sarcoma. Cancer *37*:2476–2485, 1976.

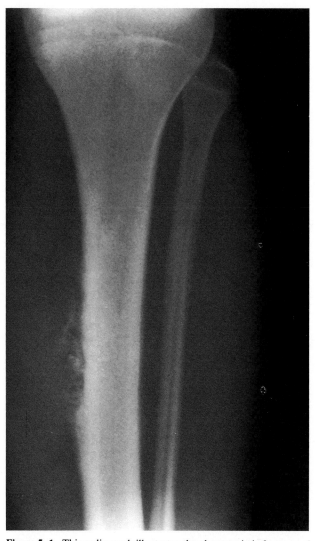

**Figure 5–1.** This radiograph illustrates the characteristic features of periosteal osteosarcoma. The tumor arises from the surface of the tibial diaphysis and is partially calcified.

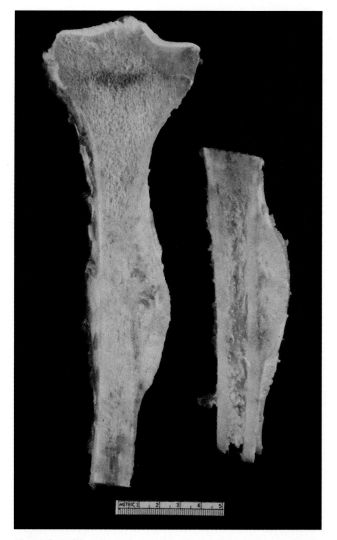

**Figure 5–2.** The bisected gross specimen shown in Figure 5–1 illustrates the surface nature of periosteal osteosarcoma as it affects the tibial diaphysis, the most commonly affected bone. Grossly no visible tumor should be evident in the medullary portion of the affected bone.

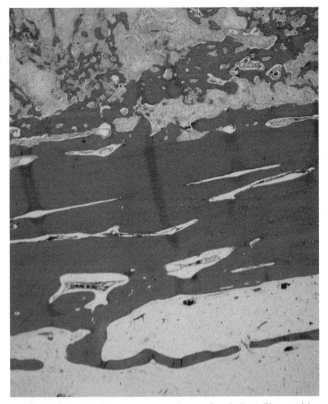

**Figure 5–3.** Periosteal osteosarcoma is a surface lesion of bone without medullary involvement. This photomicrograph at low magnification shows the uninvolved medullary region and the surface chondroblastic tumor.

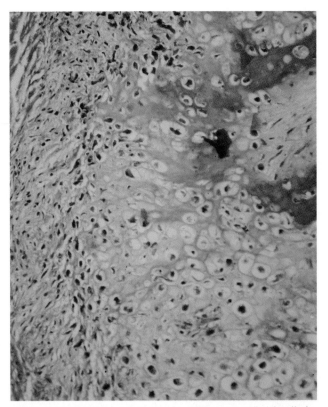

**Figure 5–5.** At higher magnification, osteoid is identified focally in the lesion. The focal nature of the osteoid production results in confusion of this tumor with periosteal chondrosarcoma and periosteal chondroma.

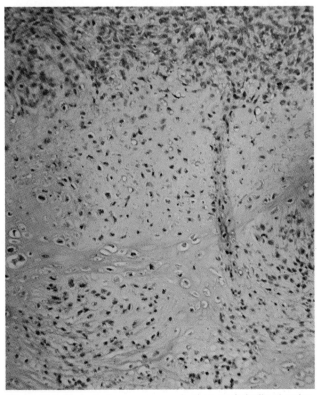

**Figure 5–4.** Periosteal osteosarcoma is characteristically chondroblastic, as shown in this photomicrograph. At the periphery of the chondroid islands a "condensation" of spindle cells is visible.

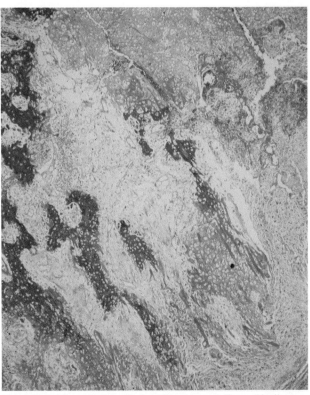

**Figure 5–6.** The radiating spicules of bone seen radiographicaly correspond to the bone seen at low magnification in this photomicrograph. Such osteoid frequently traverses the lesion perpendicularly to the underlying cortical bone.

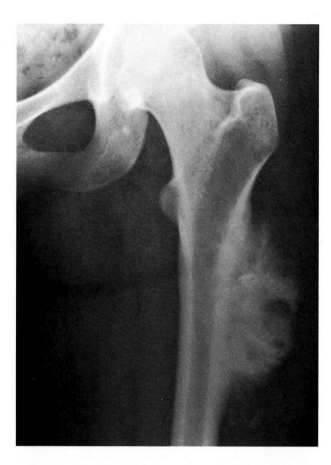

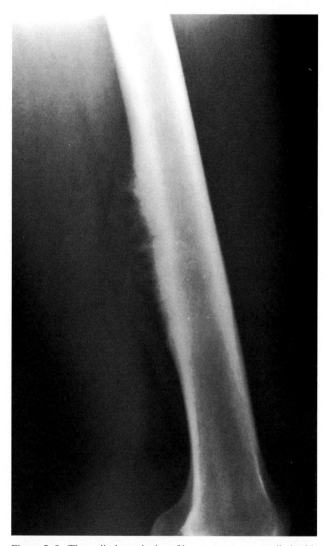

**Figure 5–7.** The femoral diaphysis is a common location for periosteal osteosarcoma, as is shown in this radiograph. This tumor is large and shows the spiculated mineralization commonly identified in periosteal osteosarcoma.

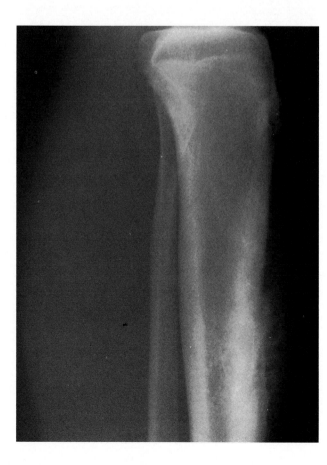

**Figure 5–8.** The radiating spicules of bone are seen centrally in this periosteal osteosarcoma of the lower femoral diaphysis. An unmineralized soft tissue mass is seen at the periphery of the tumor.

**Figure 5–9.** The most common location for periosteal osteosarcoma is the tibial diaphysis, as is shown in this radiograph. The cortex in this case is thickened, but the underlying medulla is uninvolved.

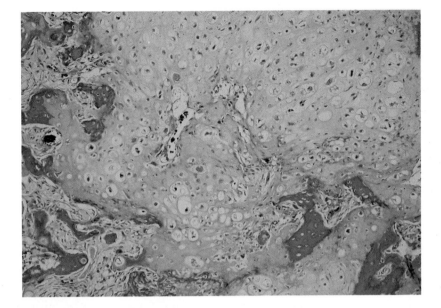

**Figure 5–10.** Chondroid matrix commonly predominates in periosteal osteosarcoma. However, osteoid is identifiable at the periphery of the chondroid zones in this photomicrograph.

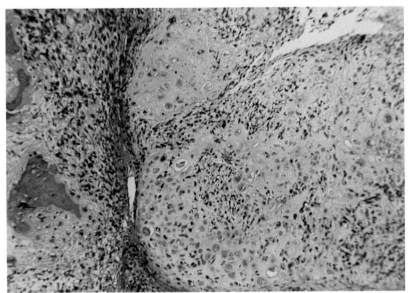

**Figure 5–11.** These tumors frequently show the lobulation that is commonly seen in cartilaginous tumors. However, at the periphery of the lobules the tumor shows greater cellularity and atypia than is evident in chondrosarcomas.

**Figure 5–12.** Some periosteal osteosarcomas show greater regions of spindle cell proliferation, as in this case. With such lesions the differential diagnosis is between high-grade surface osteosarcoma and periosteal osteosarcoma.

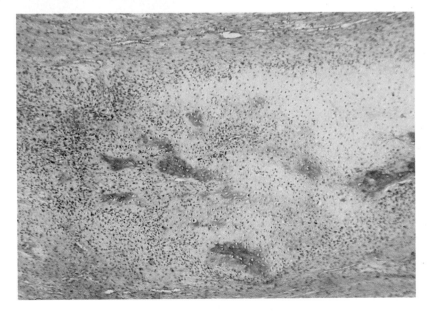

# CHAPTER 6

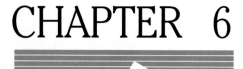

# High-grade Surface Osteosarcoma

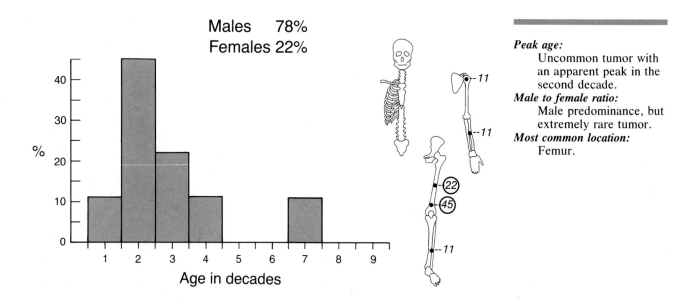

Males 78%
Females 22%

%

40

30

20

10

0

1 2 3 4 5 6 7 8 9

Age in decades

--11

--11

22
45

--11

**Peak age:**
Uncommon tumor with an apparent peak in the second decade.
**Male to female ratio:**
Male predominance, but extremely rare tumor.
**Most common location:**
Femur.

■ **Clinical Symptoms**

1. Pain is present in the region of the tumor.
2. Swelling is noted in the region of the tumor.

■ **Clinical Signs**

1. A painful mass lesion is present.
2. The lesion may be warm.
3. Erythema may be present in the skin overlying the tumor.

■ **Major Radiographic Features**

1. A partially mineralized tumor is seen on the surface of a long bone, most commonly the femur.
2. Cortical destruction is usually apparent.
3. Periosteal new bone is often present.

■ **Radiographic Differential Diagnosis**

1. Periosteal osteosarcoma.
2. Parosteal osteosarcoma.
3. Periosteal chondrosarcoma.

■ **Pathologic Features**

*Gross*

1. The tumor is situated on the surface of the affected bone and may extend into the cortex, but should lack significant medullary involvement.
2. Consistency of the lesional tissue varies from firm to soft and in general resembles that of ordinary osteosarcoma.
3. Chondroid differentiation consisting of bluish-white lobules of tissue may be grossly evident.

*Microscopic*

1. At low magnification these tumors vary from region to region.
2. Zones of chondroid differentiation, zones of spindle cell proliferation, and zones containing dense osteoid may be identified.
3. At higher magnification, marked nuclear and cytologic pleomorphism—identical with that seen

with conventional high-grade intramedullary osteosarcoma—is present.
4. Mitotic activity is usually brisk.
5. Lace-like osteoid production should be identifiable.
6. Minimal amounts of tumor may be present in the medullary cavity.

## ■ Pathologic Differential Diagnosis

Benign lesions:
1. Myositis ossificans (heterotopic ossification).
Malignant lesions:
1. Periosteal osteosarcoma.
2. Conventional osteosarcoma with prominent soft tissue extension.
3. Parosteal osteosarcoma.

## ■ Treatment

**Primary Modality:** similar to conventional osteosarcoma—limb-saving resection with a wide margin (if feasible) or amputation (if necessary) to obtain a wide margin. Neoadjuvant polychemotherapy protocols are utilized, similar to conventional osteosarcoma.

**Other Possible Approaches:** radiotherapy for surgically inaccessible lesions and aggressive thoracotomy for pulmonary metastases.

## References

Schajowicz F, McGuire MH, Araujo ES, et al: Osteosarcomas arising on the surfaces of long bones. J Bone Joint Surg 70A:555–564, 1988.

Wold LE, Unni KK, Beabout JW, and Dahlin DC: High-grade surface osteosarcomas. Am J Surg Pathol 8:181–186, 1984.

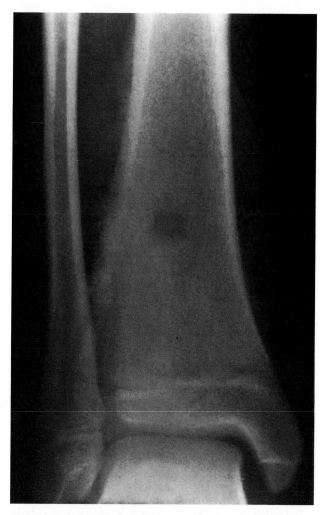

**Figure 6–1.** This radiograph illustrates the features of a high-grade surface osteosarcoma of the diametaphyseal region of the lower tibia. Note the matrix ossification projecting lateral to and over the tibia. The cortical defect evident is due to prior biopsy.

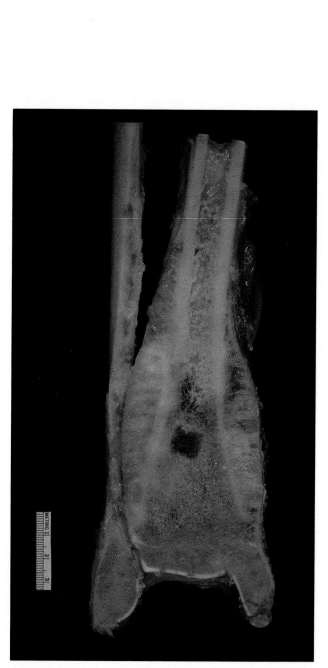

**Figure 6–2.** This gross photograph illustrates the appearance of a high-grade surface osteosarcoma involving the distal tibia. No medullary tumor is present; the defect at the center of the distal tibia represents a prior biopsy site.

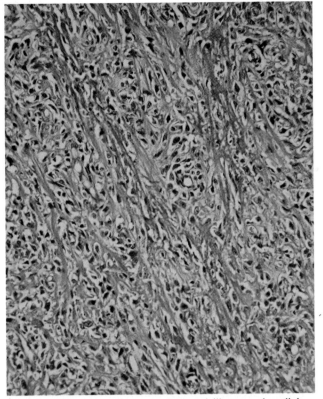

**Figure 6–3.** This low-power photomicrograph illustrates the cellular, anaplastic nature of high-grade surface osteosarcomas. The histologic spectrum for this subtype of osteosarcoma is identical with the usual intramedullary-type osteosarcoma.

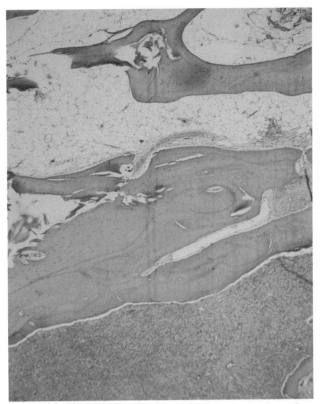

**Figure 6–5.** Although the cortical bone may be eroded in the surface variants of osteosarcoma, medullary involvement is lacking, as is illustrated in this example of a high-grade surface osteosarcoma of the tibia.

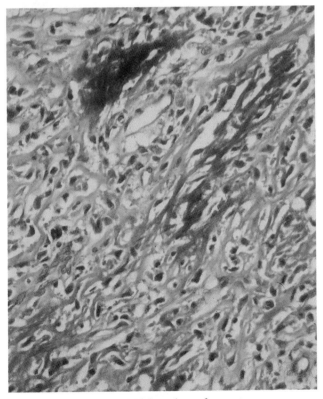

**Figure 6–4.** Examples of high-grade surface osteosarcoma may show little osteoid, as is illustrated in this photomicrograph.

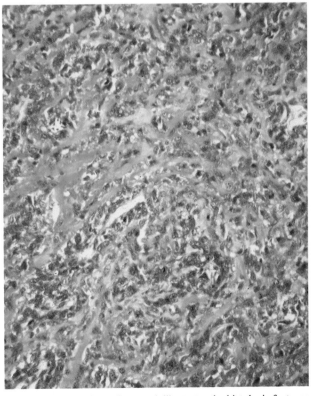

**Figure 6–6.** This photomicrograph illustrates the histologic features of a high-grade surface osteosarcoma treated initially with limb salvage. The tumor metastasized to the pelvis, and the patient died from further metastatic disease.

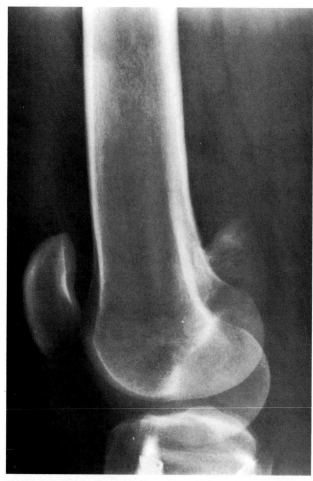

**Figure 6–7.** This radiograph illustrates a high-grade surface osteosarcoma arising from the posterior surface of the distal femoral metaphysis. Note the radiating bone spicules extending posteriorly into the sizable soft tissue mass. The medulla of the femur appears uninvolved.

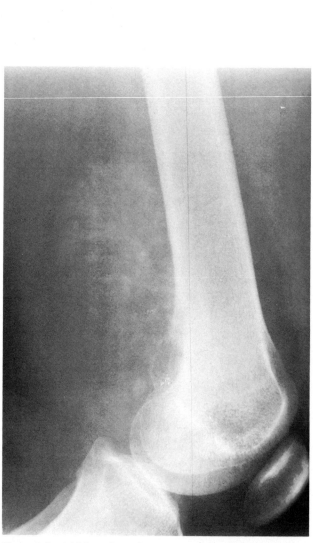

**Figure 6–8.** A high-grade surface osteosarcoma of the distal femur is shown in this radiograph. Note the large ossified soft tissue mass posterior to the femur. The tumor affects only the superficial cortical bone.

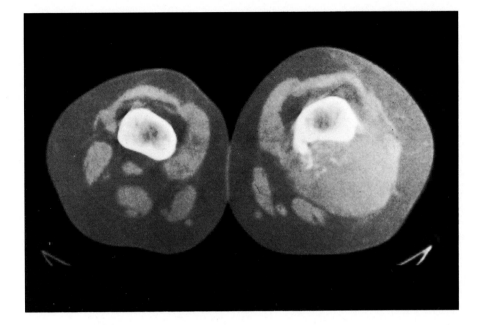

**Figure 6–9.** The CT scan of the same case verifies the surface location of the tumor, delineating the soft tissue mass and confirming the absence of a medullary component of the lesion.

# CHAPTER 7

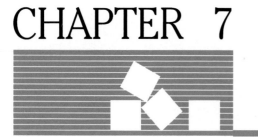

# Telangiectatic Osteosarcoma

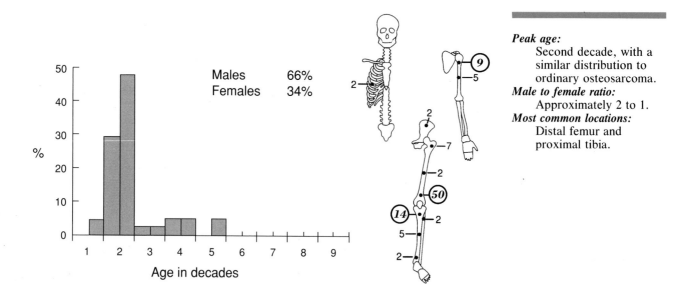

Males 66%
Females 34%

**Peak age:**
Second decade, with a similar distribution to ordinary osteosarcoma.
**Male to female ratio:**
Approximately 2 to 1.
**Most common locations:**
Distal femur and proximal tibia.

■ **Clinical Symptoms**

1. Pain is present.
2. Swelling is noted in the region of the tumor.

■ **Clinical Signs**

1. A tender mass lesion is noted.
2. Occasional pathologic fracture may be seen.

■ **Major Radiographic Features**

1. The tumor is metaphyseal in location and large in size.
2. There is considerable medullary and cortical bone destruction.
3. The lesion is purely lytic and poorly marginated.
4. Periosteal new bone and soft tissue mass are common.

■ **Radiographic Differential Diagnosis**

1. Ordinary osteosarcoma.
2. Fibrosarcoma.
3. Malignant fibrous histiocytoma.
4. Aneurysmal bone cyst.

■ **Pathologic Features**

*Gross*

1. Lesional tissue is hemorrhagic.
2. Firm, fleshy areas are not identifiable in this tumor.
3. Lesional tissue is arranged in delicate strands coursing through the blood clot.

*Microscopic*

1. At low magnification the features are similar to aneurysmal bone cyst.

2. Septa traverse and surround blood-filled spaces.
3. At higher magnification the cytologic features show that the mononuclear cells are pleomorphic.
4. Benign multinucleated giant cells are almost uniformly present.
5. Osteoid production is generally focal and minimal.

## ■ Pathologic Differential Diagnosis

Benign lesions:
1. Aneurysmal bone cyst.
Malignant lesions:
1. Malignancy in giant cell tumor (malignant giant cell tumor).
2. Hemangioendothelial sarcoma.

## ■ Treatment

**Primary Modality:** as in conventional osteosarcoma, surgical ablation by amputation or limb-saving resection. Multidrug chemotherapy in a neoadjuvant setting is most commonly used.

**Other Possible Approaches:** radiation therapy for lesions in inaccessible sites.

## References

Huvos AG, Rosen G, Bretsky SS, and Butler A: Telangiectatic osteogenic sarcoma: a clinicopathologic study of 124 patients. Cancer *49*:1679–1689, 1982.

Matsuno T, Unni KK, McLeod RA, and Dahlin DC: Telangiectatic osteogenic sarcoma. Cancer *38*:2538–2547, 1976.

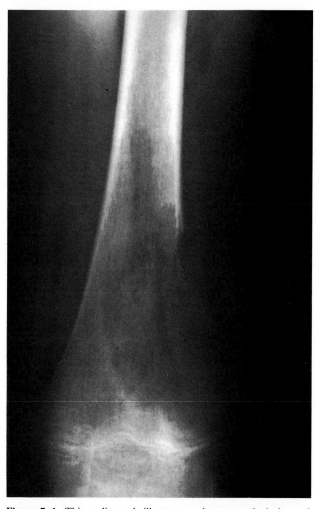

**Figure 7–1.** This radiograph illustrates a large, purely lytic, and poorly marginated tumor in the distal femoral metaphysis. Considerable destruction of the medullary and cortical bone is evident with associated soft tissue extension. The purely lytic appearance is characteristic of telangiectatic osteosarcoma.

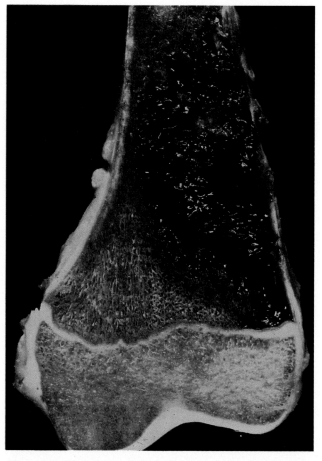

**Figure 7–2.** The gross pathologic features of telangiectatic osteosarcoma are illustrated in this photograph. The lesion is invariably hemorrhagic and may be quite cystic. Both grossly and microscopically it may be mistaken for an aneurysmal bone cyst.

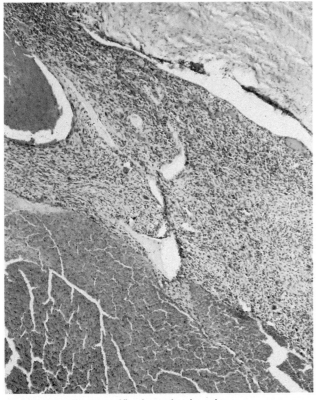

**Figure 7–3.** At low magnification, telangiectatic osteosarcoma contains large blood-filled spaces similar to the pattern seen in an aneurysmal bone cyst.

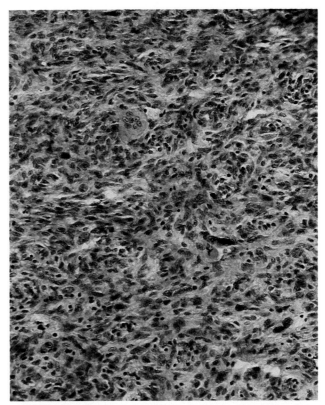

**Figure 7–5.** Solid areas of the tumor should be only a minor component of this tumor. Abnormal mitotic figures and benign giant cells are commonly found.

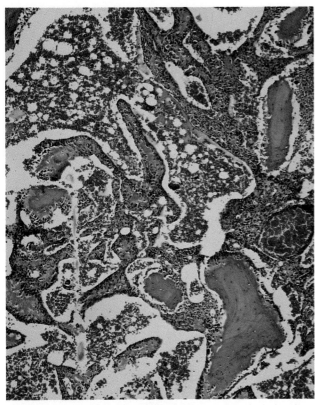

**Figure 7–4.** This photomicrograph shows the edge of a lesion demonstrating permeation of medullary bone. The bony trabeculae are normal and are not produced by the tumor.

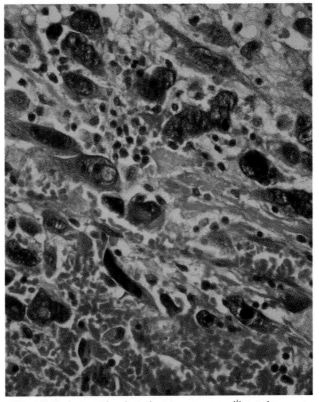

**Figure 7–6.** A rare telangiectatic osteosarcoma will not show septa and spaces but instead will be composed of very pleomorphic-appearing cells within a blood clot.

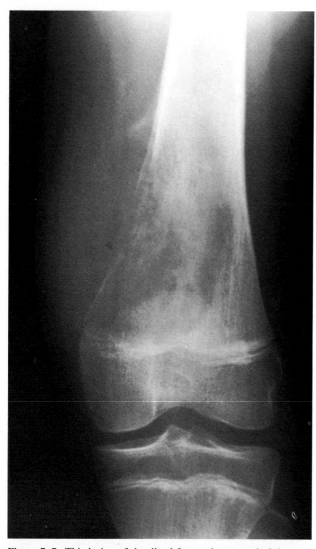

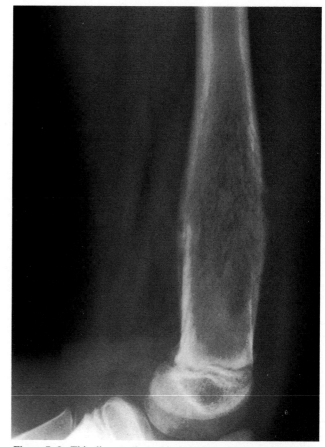

**Figure 7–8.** This diametaphyseal lytic lesion with poor margination and a permeative growth pattern also represents a telangiectatic osteosarcoma.

**Figure 7–7.** This lesion of the distal femur shows cortical destruction, Codman's triangle, and an associated soft tissue mass. These features support a high-grade malignant diagnosis. The purely lytic nature of the lesion is compatible with the diagnosis of telangiectatic osteosarcoma, which it proved to be histologically.

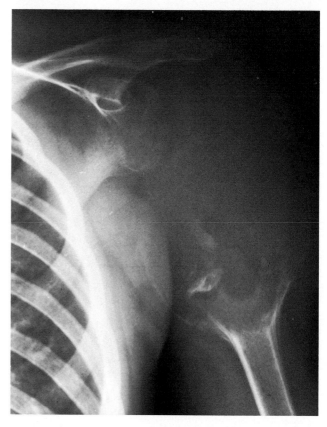

**Figure 7–9.** This proximal humeral lesion shows the "blown-out" appearance occasionally seen with an aneurysmal bone cyst. This lesion was confirmed histologically to be a telangiectatic osteosarcoma. The overlap of radiographic and histologic features of aneurysmal bone cyst and telangiectatic osteosarcoma makes these lesions particularly difficult diagnostic problems for the pathologist.

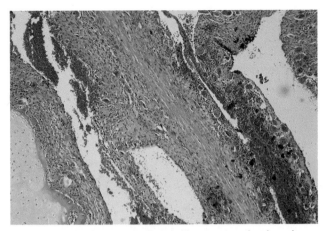

**Figure 7–10.** This photomicrograph illustrates a telangiectatic osteosarcoma that markedly simulates an aneurysmal bone cyst. Benign multinucleated giant cells are present, and some of the septa are fibrotic and hypocellular.

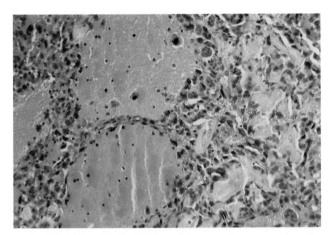

**Figure 7–11.** Careful examination of the septa is necessary in order to identify the cytologic atypia, as shown in this photomicrograph, which separates telangiectatic osteosarcoma from an aneurysmal bone cyst.

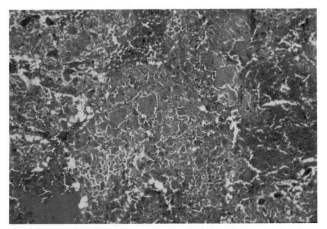

**Figure 7–12.** When multinucleated giant cells are numerous, as in this case, a telangiectatic osteosarcoma may focally resemble a giant cell tumor.

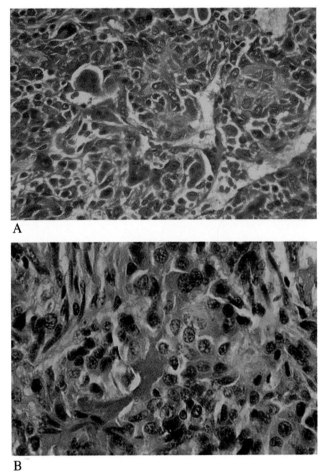

A

B

**Figure 7–13.** At high magnification, the cytologic atypia of the mononuclear cells illustrated in A and B distinguishes telangiectatic osteosarcoma from a giant cell tumor. Osteoid production (B) should be minimal.

# CHAPTER 8

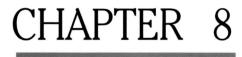

# Low-grade Central Osteosarcoma

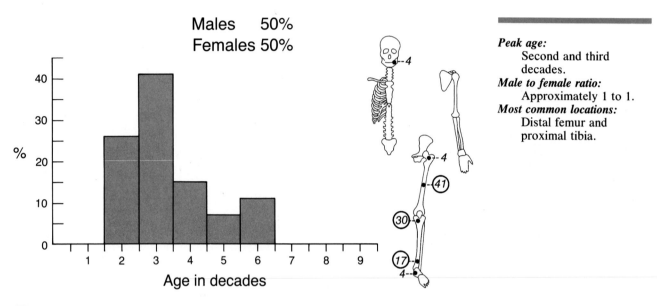

Males    50%
Females 50%

Age in decades

**Peak age:**
    Second and third
    decades.
**Male to female ratio:**
    Approximately 1 to 1.
**Most common locations:**
    Distal femur and
    proximal tibia.

## ■ Clinical Symptoms

1. Pain is a common presenting complaint.
2. A swelling is almost never noted.

## ■ Clinical Signs

1. Usually no specific signs are elicited on physical examination.

## ■ Major Radiographic Features

1. Medullary lesions usually extend to the end of the bone.
2. The tumor is poorly marginated and large.
3. Most are trabeculated or sclerotic.
4. Periosteal new bone and soft tissue mass are usually absent.
5. The overall appearance may suggest benignity, with only a small region showing features that suggest malignancy.

## ■ Radiographic Differential Diagnosis

1. Fibrous dysplasia.
2. Giant cell tumor.

3. Ordinary osteosarcoma.
4. Fibrosarcoma.
5. Malignant fibrous histiocytoma.

## ■ Pathologic Features

### Gross

1. These lesions are firm and fibrous, lacking the "fleshy" appearance of high-grade sarcomas.
2. A gritty quality somewhat like fibrous dysplasia may be noted.
3. The tumor is most commonly confined to the medullary cavity without an associated soft tissue mass; however, the cortex is destroyed, at least focally.

### Microscopic

1. The low-magnification appearance of this tumor mimics that of fibrous dysplasia.
2. The lesional tissue is composed of disordered or irregular bony trabeculae, between which is a hypocellular spindle cell proliferation (the pat-

tern is essentially identical with that seen in parosteal osteosarcoma).
3. At higher magnification the spindle cells show little pleomorphism or anaplasia, and mitotic activity is extremely low. The spindle cells may be arranged in a "herring bone" or a storiform pattern.
4. The osteoid appears "normalized" as in parosteal osteosarcoma.

### ■ Pathologic Differential Diagnosis

Benign lesions:
1. Fibrous dysplasia
2. Osteofibrous dysplasia
Malignant lesions:
1. Osteosarcoma, ordinary intramedullary type.
2. Parosteal osteosarcoma (if location is not considered).

### ■ Treatment

**Primary Modality:** surgical resection with a wide margin and skeletal reconstruction with osteochondral allograft, custom prosthesis, or resection arthrodesis, depending on the location of the lesion and the patient's needs.

**Other Possible Approaches:** amputation if an adequately wide margin cannot be achieved by surgical resection. Chemotherapy is not indicated unless there has been recurrence and "dedifferentiation" of the tumor.

### References

Unni KK, Dahlin DC, McLeod RA, and Pritchard DJ: Intraosseous well-differentiated osteosarcoma. Cancer 40:1337–1347, 1977.

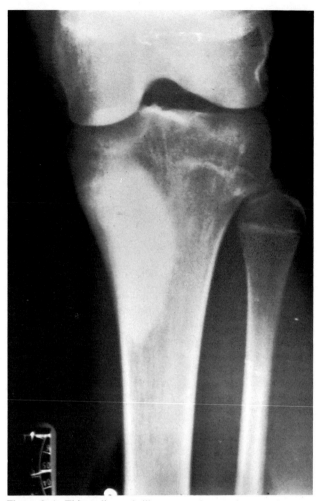

**Figure 8–1.** This radiograph illustrates a low-grade central osteo-sarcoma of the medulla of the upper tibia. The lesion is densely sclerotic.

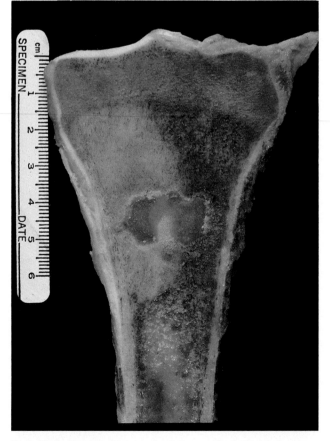

**Figure 8–2.** A gross photograph of the proximal tibial lesion seen in Figure 8–1 shows the homogeneous nature of most low-grade central osteosarcomas. The central defect is the biopsy site. These tumors are frequently gritty when cut.

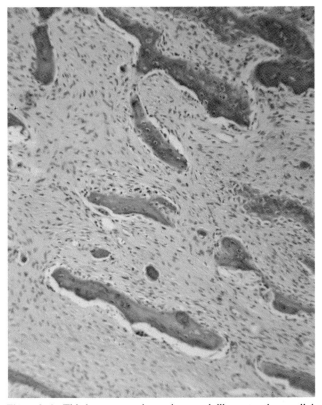

**Figure 8–3.** This low-power photomicrograph illustrates the parallel arrangement of bony trabeculae that can be seen in low-grade central osteosarcomas. This appearance is nearly identical with that of parosteal osteosarcoma.

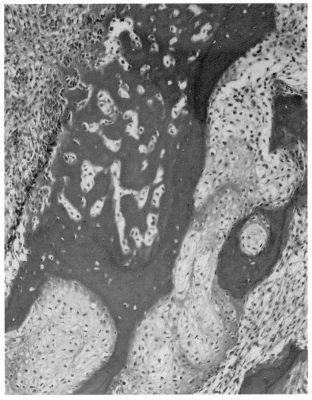

**Figure 8–5.** The osteoid produced by low-grade central osteosarcoma may grow in an appositional manner onto pre-existing bony trabeculae.

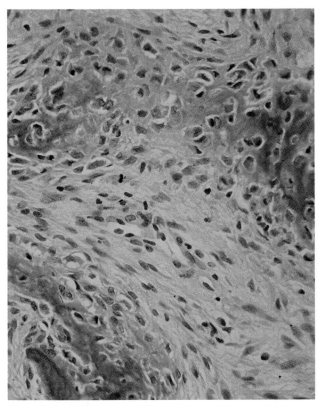

**Figure 8–4.** At higher magnification, low-grade central osteosarcomas show minimal cytologic atypia. The lesions are also less cellular than conventional osteosarcomas.

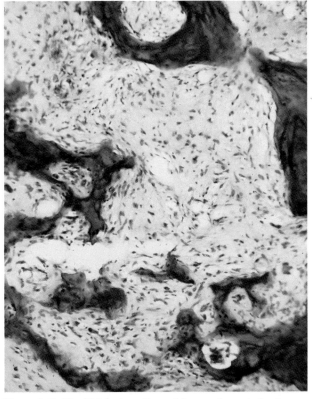

**Figure 8–6.** The histologic pattern of low-grade central osteosarcoma may also mimic that seen in fibrous dysplasia, as is illustrated in this photomicrograph.

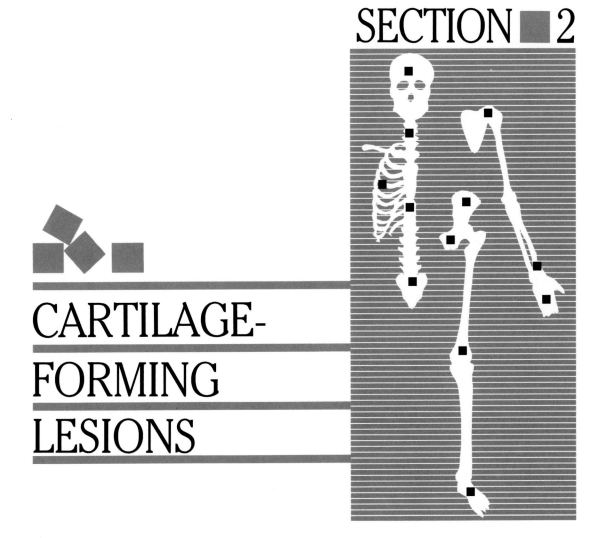

# SECTION ■ 2

# CARTILAGE-FORMING LESIONS

# CHAPTER 9

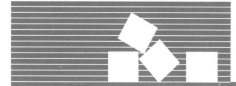

# Osteochondroma

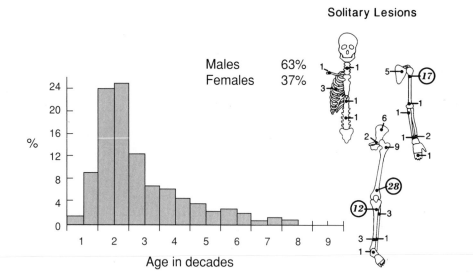

Solitary Lesions

Males 63%
Females 37%

*Peak age:*
Second decade.
*Male to female ratio:*
1.7 to 1.
*Most common location:*
Distal femur.

■ **Clinical Symptoms**

1. A mass lesion, usually of long duration, is present.
2. Pain may result secondary to impingement on an overlying structure or to bursa formation.
3. Pain may rarely be related to fracture through the stalk of a pedunculated lesion.

■ **Clinical Signs**

1. A palpable mass is noted.

■ **Major Radiographic Features**

1. Peripheral bone projection or growth is present.
2. There is continuity of the cortical and cancellous bone from the underlying parent bone to the lesion.

3. There is flaring of the metaphysis of the affected bone.

■ **Radiographic Differential Diagnosis**

1. Parosteal osteochondromatous proliferation.
2. Parosteal osteosarcoma.
3. Myositis ossificans.

■ **Pathologic Features**

*Gross*

1. The cut surface of the lesion shows a thin (usually less than 1 cm), smooth, translucent, bluish cartilaginous cap.
2. Cancellous bone underlies the cartilaginous cap.
3. Lesions may be pedunculated or sessile with a broad base.

*Microscopic*

1. The thin cartilaginous cap mimics the appearance of an epiphyseal plate with maturation via enchondral ossification to regular bony trabeculae.
2. At higher magnification the chondrocytes are seen to be arranged in a linear fashion, and the nuclei lack pleomorphism, nuclear hyperchromasia, and binucleation.
3. The intertrabecular space is filled with fatty or hematopoietic marrow.

## ■ Pathologic Differential Diagnosis

Benign lesions:
1. Parosteal osteocartilaginous proliferation.
Malignant lesions:
1. Parosteal osteosarcoma.
2. Chondrosarcoma arising in an osteochondroma.

## ■ Treatment

**Primary Modality:** Treatment is individualized depending on clinical circumstances. Most lesions, either solitary or multiple, are simply observed.

**Other Possible Approaches:** If the lesion is symptomatic or cosmetically disfiguring, surgical excision at the base of the exostosis is carried out to remove the entire cartilage cap.

## References

Borges AM, Huvos AB, and Smith J: Bursa formation and synovial chondrometaplasia associated with osteochondromas. Am J Clin Pathol 75:648–653, 1981.

Landon GC, Johnson KA, and Dahlin DC: Subungual exostoses. J Bone Joint Surg 61A:256–259, 1979.

Nora FE, Dahlin DC, and Beabout JW: Bizarre parosteal osteochondromatous proliferations of the hands and feet. Am J Surg Pathol 7:245–250, 1983.

Shapiro F, Simon S, and Glimcher MJ: Hereditary multiple exostoses: anthropometric, roentgenographic, and clinical aspects. J Bone Joint Surg 61A:815–824, 1979.

Solomon L: Hereditary multiple exostosis. Am J Hum Genet 16:351–363, 1964.

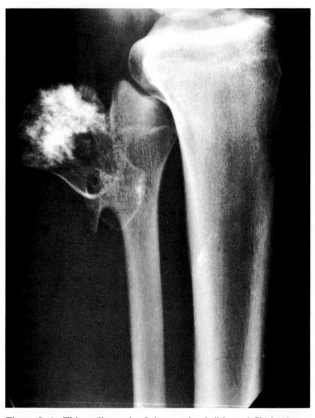

**Figure 9–1.** This radiograph of the proximal tibia and fibula shows a heavily mineralized osteochondroma projecting posteriorly from the upper fibular metaphysis. The continuity of the cortical and cancellous bone of the fibula with the lesion is characteristic of osteochondroma.

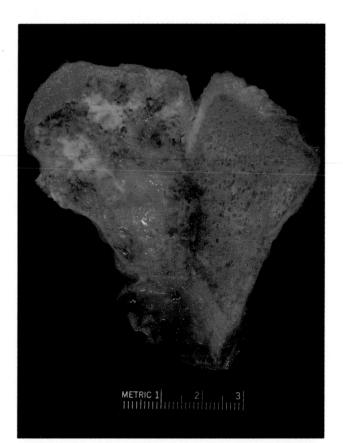

**Figure 9–2.** Grossly, the resected osteochondroma illustrated in Figure 9–1 shows a cartilaginous cap with regions of extensive calcification (white areas) corresponding to the heavily mineralized regions seen radiographically. The thickness of the cartilage cap is a gross pathologic feature that helps to identify lesions that should be carefully assessed histologically for malignant transformation of the cartilage.

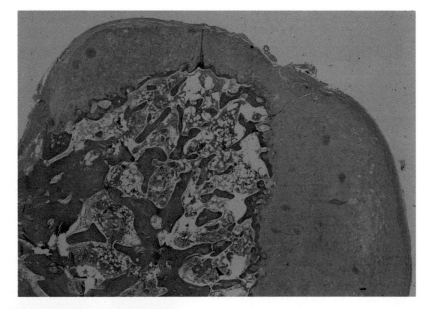

**Figure 9–3.** At low magnification osteochondromas show a well-circumscribed periphery. The hyaline cartilage matures into the underlying trabecular bone.

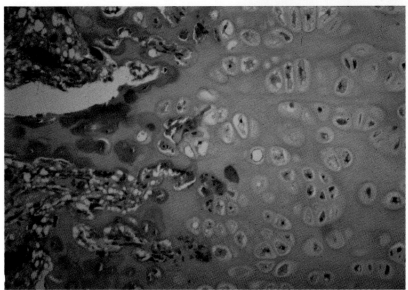

**Figure 9–4.** At higher magnification the transition between the cartilage and the osseous trabeculae is identical with a normal growth plate, with columns of chondrocytes and ossification of the matrix material.

**Figure 9–5.** At high magnification the chondrocytes in the cartilage cap have small, dark-staining nuclei that lack cytologic atypia.

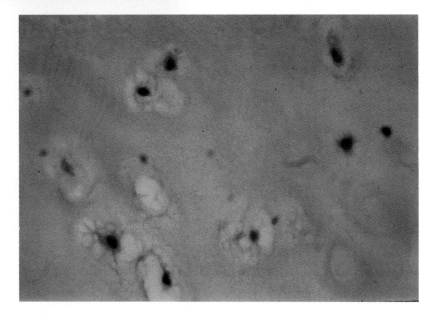

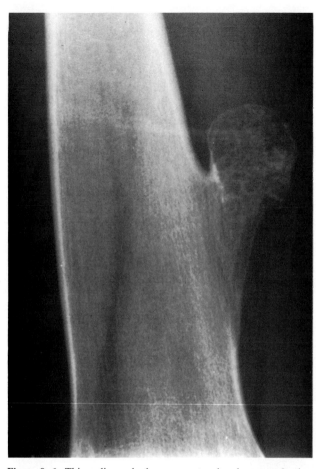

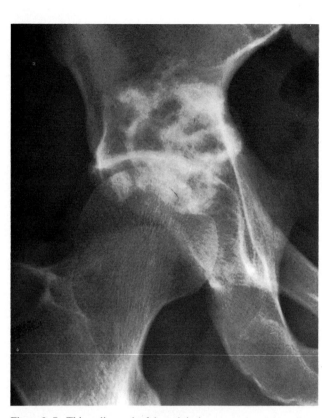

**Figure 9–6.** This radiograph shows an osteochondroma projecting from the lower femur. The continuity of cortical and cancellous bone is evident. In general, pedunculated osteochondromas point away from the closest joint.

**Figure 9–7.** This radiograph of the pelvis demonstrates a mineralized lesion above the acetabulum. Flat-bone osteochondromas such as this may be difficult to localize and characterize with plain x-rays; CT scans are particularly helpful in this situation.

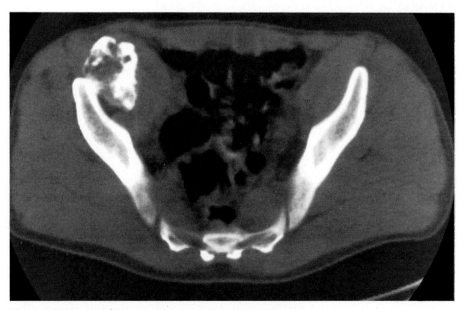

**Figure 9–8.** An axial CT scan of the patient in Figure 9–7 demonstrates the typical appearance of an osteochondroma projecting from the anterior iliac bone.

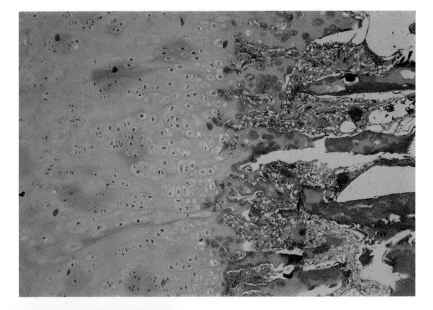

**Figure 9–9.** Between the osseous trabeculae of an osteochondroma is fatty or hematopoietic marrow, as is shown in this photomicrograph. In contrast, parosteal osteosarcoma, which may also have a cartilaginous cap, has a spindle-cell proliferation between the "normalized trabeculae" of bone.

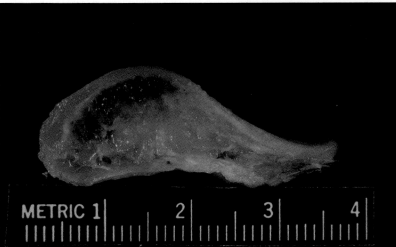

**Figure 9–10.** This osteochondroma of the distal femur shows the thin cartilage cap and the continuity of the cortical and cancellous bone that characterize the lesion.

**Figure 9–11.** Subungual exostoses (as shown in this photograph) share some gross and microscopic features with osteochondromas.

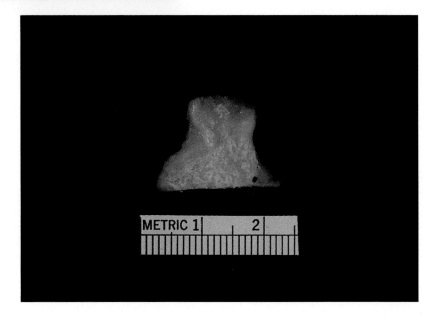

# CHAPTER 10

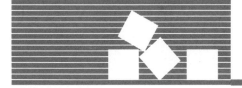

# Chondroma

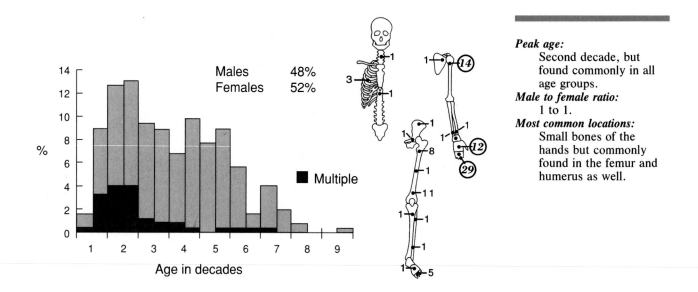

Males 48%
Females 52%

■ Multiple

% — Age in decades

**Peak age:**
Second decade, but
found commonly in all
age groups.
**Male to female ratio:**
1 to 1.
**Most common locations:**
Small bones of the
hands but commonly
found in the femur and
humerus as well.

■ **Clinical Symptoms**

1. The majority are asymptomatic.
2. Pain is rarely a presenting complaint but may be
   present in patients with pathologic fractures.
   This is commonly the case with lesions of the
   small bones. If pain exists in the absence of
   pathologic fracture, the suspicion of a low-grade
   chondrosarcoma should be raised.

■ **Clinical Signs**

1. Frequently chondromas are diagnosed incidentally on radiographic examination.
2. Chondromas are frequently "hot" on bone scan
   and may be incidentally identified in this way as
   well.

■ **Major Radiographic Features**

1. The lesion is medullary in location.

2. The features are benign, showing sharp margination and expansion of the affected bone.
3. Punctate calcification frequently is present.
4. Multiple lesions may be seen.

■ **Radiographic Differential Diagnosis**

1. Bone infarct.
2. Chondrosarcoma.

■ **Pathologic Features**

*Gross*

1. Lesional tissue is characteristically translucent
   and blue-gray in color.
2. Whitish-yellow calcific foci may be scattered
   throughout the tissue.
3. The tumors vary in consistency, but most are
   relatively firm. Myxoid foci should arouse suspicion that the tumor is a low-grade chondrosarcoma.

*Microscopic*

1. On low magnification the tumor is hypocellular and has a blue-gray aura to the cartilaginous matrix.
2. The nuclei are inconspicuous on low magnification.
3. On higher magnification the nuclei are uniform in their cytologic characteristics. Each is small, regular, and darkly stained.
4. Binucleated cells are rare.

## ■ Pathologic Differential Diagnosis

Benign lesions:
1. Fibrocartilaginous dysplasia with prominent chondroid regions.
2. The cartilage of a prominent costochondral junction.

Malignant lesions:
1. Low-grade (well differentiated) chondrosarcoma.
2. Chondroblastic osteosarcoma.

## ■ Treatment

**Primary Modality:**  A benign appearing, asymptomatic enchondroma that is not structurally weakening the bone warrants observation.

**Other Possible Approaches:**  If the lesion is symptomatic, curettage and bone grafting usually are curative. If there is an associated pathologic fracture, curettage and grafting should be delayed until the fracture has healed and the continuity of the bone has been restored.

## References

Bauer TW, Dorfman HD, and Lathan JT Jr: Periosteal chondroma: a clinicopathologic study of 23 cases. Am J Surg Pathol 6:631–637, 1982.

Boriani S, Bacchini P, Bertoni F, and Campanacci M: Periosteal chondroma: a review of twenty cases. J Bone Joint Surg 65A:205–212, 1983.

DeSantos LA, and Spjut HJ: Periosteal chondroma: a radiographic spectrum. Skeletal Radiol 6:15–20, 1981.

**Figure 10–1.** This radiograph shows an enchondroma in its most common location, a phalanx of the hand. The lesion is well marginated and expansile. The typical punctate calcification of a cartilaginous lesion is present.

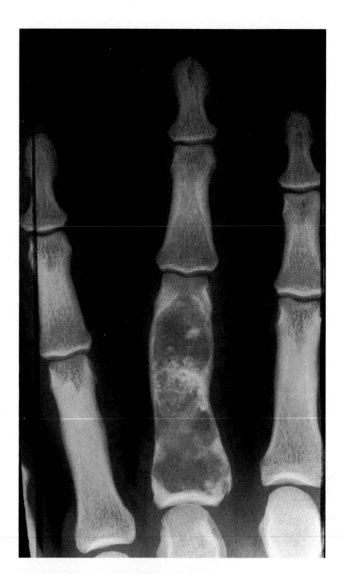

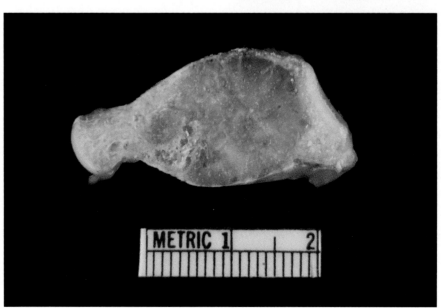

**Figure 10–2.** The gross appearance of hyaline cartilage lesions is shown in this photograph of a phalangeal chondroma. The lesion is well circumscribed, glistening, and gray-white in color. The small bones may be expanded by such a lesion, as is illustrated in this case.

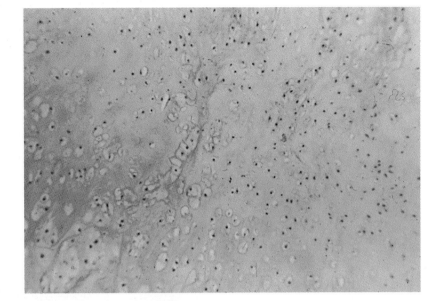

**Figure 10–3.** At low magnification, hyaline cartilage lesions are blue-gray in color. Benign lesions are hypocellular, as is illustrated in this photomicrograph of a chondroma involving the femoral diaphysis.

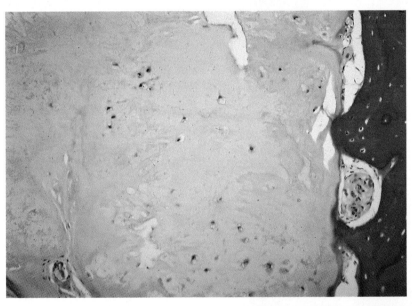

**Figure 10–4.** The periphery of a chondroma is well circumscribed both grossly and microscopically, as is illustrated in this photomicrograph of a fibular chondroma. The lesion does not show significant endosteal erosion.

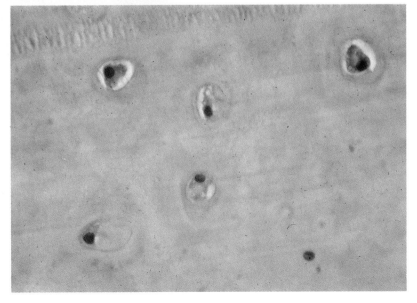

**Figure 10–5.** At higher magnification the cytologic features of the chondrocytes are apparent. In a chondroma the nuclei are uniformly small and darkly stained. Although binucleated cells may be seen occasionally, they are not common.

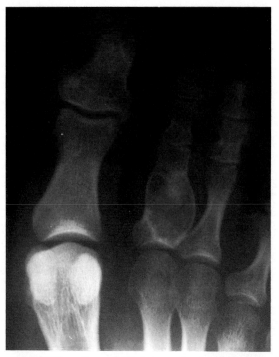

**Figure 10–6.** This radiograph illustrates a chondroma involving the middle phalanx of the second toe. The lesion expands the affected bone, is calcified, and shows a sclerotic margin.

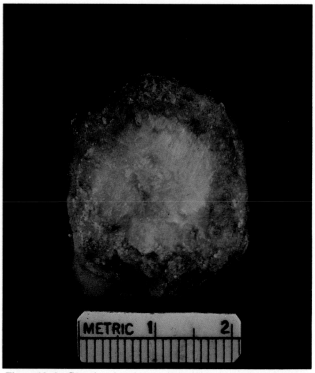

**Figure 10–8.** Grossly, chondromas in long-bone locations are no different from those involving the small bones of the hands and feet. This chondroma of the upper fibula shows the well-marginated, glistening, gray-white aura of a hyaline cartilage tumor.

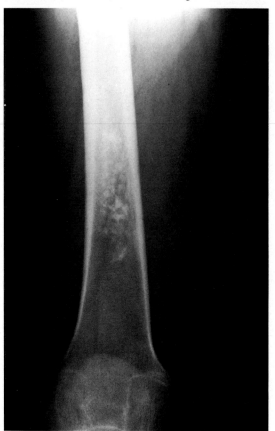

**Figure 10–7.** When chondromas involve the long bones, the lesions generally show an intramedullary collection of stippled calcification. Ring-like calcification may also be present. The endosteal surface of the affected bone does not show any irregularity. Endosteal erosion is a feature that is worrisome for a low-grade malignant cartilage tumor.

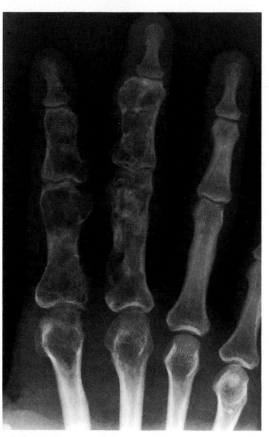

**Figure 10–9.** Multiple chondromas show the same radiographic features as solitary lesions, as is shown in this case with multiple lesions involving the small bones of the hand.

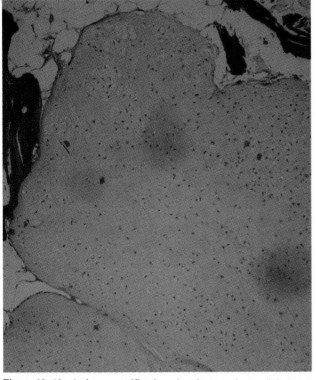

**Figure 10–10.** At low magnification chondromas show a lobulated pattern, as is illustrated in this case. Many cartilage tumors share this low-power histologic feature.

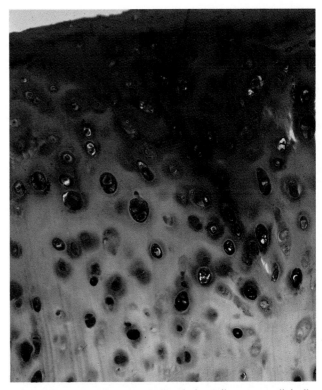

**Figure 10–12.** Prominent costochondral cartilage may clinically mimic the appearance of a neoplasm. If biopsied, a mistaken diagnosis of a cartilage tumor may be made. However, the regular and orderly appearance of the chondrocytes is a clue that the tissue represents normal anatomy rather than neoplasm.

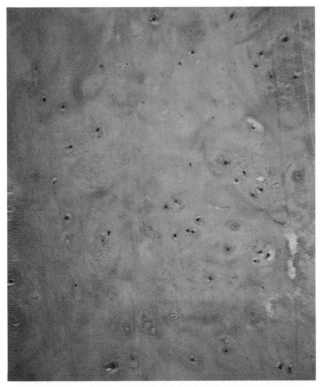

**Figure 10–11.** At low magnification the nuclei of the chondrocytes are inconspicuous, appearing as small dark dots, as is shown in this example of a chondroma involving the distal femur in an adult male.

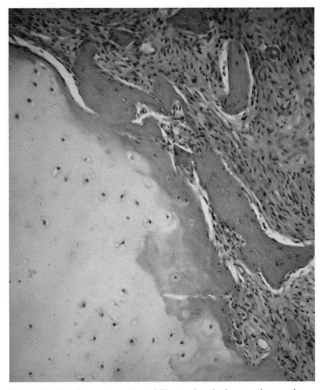

**Figure 10–13.** Some examples of fibrous dysplasia may show a chondroid component and thus be mistaken for a cartilage tumor. This case of fibrocartilaginous dysplasia involving the femur in a patient with Albright's syndrome shows such prominent chondroid differentiation.

# CHAPTER 11

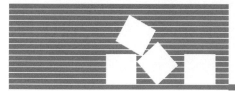

# Chondroblastoma

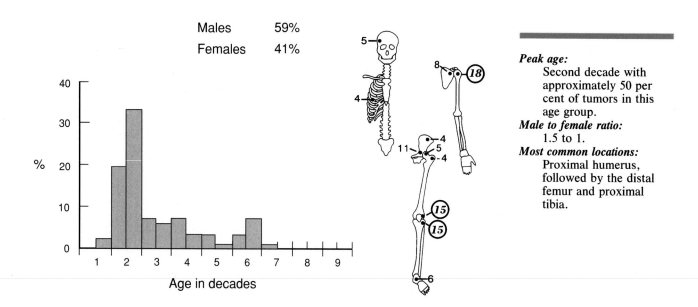

Males          59%
Females        41%

% — 40, 30, 20, 10, 0

Age in decades

**Peak age:**
    Second decade with approximately 50 per cent of tumors in this age group.
**Male to female ratio:**
    1.5 to 1.
**Most common locations:**
    Proximal humerus, followed by the distal femur and proximal tibia.

■ **Clinical Symptoms**

1. Pain localized to the region of the tumor is the most common presenting complaint and is nearly universally present.
2. The pain usually is mild to moderate in severity and may have been present from months to years at the time of diagnosis.

■ **Clinical Signs**

1. Local tenderness is usually the only finding on physical examination.
2. Muscle wasting may be present in the region of the tumor.
3. A limp may be noted since approximately 30 per cent of tumors occur around the knee joint.

■ **Major Radiographic Features**

1. The lesion is located in the epiphysis or an apophysis.

2. It is small and has sharp margins.
3. A sclerotic rim and expansion of the affected bone are commonly seen.
4. Matrix calcification is present in 25 per cent of cases.
5. The lesion may cross an open physis.

■ **Radiographic Differential Diagnosis**

1. Giant cell tumor.
2. Avascular necrosis.
3. Aneurysmal bone cyst.
4. Clear cell chondrosarcoma.

■ **Pathologic Features**

*Gross*

1. Lesional tissue is usually grayish-pink.
2. Only rarely is a grossly discernible chondroid matrix present.

3. Calcific foci may be present within curetted fragments of tissue.
4. Secondary aneurysmal bone cyst may be present, resulting in a grossly hemorrhagic or cystic specimen.

### Microscopic

1. With low magnification, multinucleated giant cells are seen scattered randomly through a "sea" of mononuclear cells, resulting in an appearance superficially resembling that of giant cell tumor.
2. Fibrochondroid islands, pinkish-blue in color, are scattered randomly through the lesional tissue.
3. Calcification may take the form of a "chicken wire" pattern or may consist of larger masses.
4. With high magnification the nuclei of the mononuclear (chondroblastic) component of the tumor are seen to be homogeneous and oval and to contain a longitudinal groove, resulting in a cytologic appearance similar to that of histiocytosis X (Langerhans' cell granulomatosis).
5. Mitotic figures, although not numerous, can be found in all cases.

### ■ Pathologic Differential Diagnosis

Benign lesions:
1. Chondromyxoid fibroma.
2. Giant cell tumor.
3. Histiocytosis X.
4. Aneurysmal bone cyst.
Malignant lesions:
1. Clear cell chondrosarcoma.
2. Chondroblastic osteosarcoma.

### ■ Treatment

**Primary Modality:** Curettage and bone grafting is curative in more than 90 per cent of cases.

**Other Possible Approaches:** en bloc excision with a marginal margin, if the lesion is located where this can be performed without significantly compromising the neighboring joint. Occasionally, in large lesions that compromise the joint with a pathologic fracture, resection with a wide margin and reconstruction with allograft, prosthesis, or arthrodesis may be necessary. Radiation therapy should be reserved for cases not amenable to surgical excision.

### References

Dahlin DC, and Ivins JC: Benign chondroblastoma: a study of 125 cases. Cancer 30:401–413, 1972.

Huvos AG, and Marcove RC: Chondroblastoma of bone: a critical review. Clin Orthop 95:300–312, 1973.

Kyriakos M, Land VJ, Penning JL, and Parker SG: Metastatic chondroblastoma: report of a fatal case with a review of the literature on atypical, aggressive and malignant chondroblastoma. Cancer 55:1770–1789, 1985.

McLeod RA, and Beabout JW: The roentgenographic features of chondroblastoma. Am J Roentgenol 118:464–471, 1973.

Roberts PF, and Taylor JG: Multifocal benign chondroblastomas: report of a case. Hum Pathol 11:296–298, 1980.

**Figure 11–1.** This radiograph shows a well-marginated lytic chondroblastoma located eccentrically in the distal femur. The knee region is the most common location for chondroblastoma, and this lesion involves the epiphysis, as is nearly always the case with chondroblastoma. The tumor also extends to involve the metaphysis.

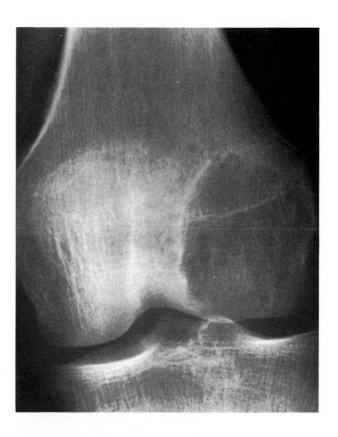

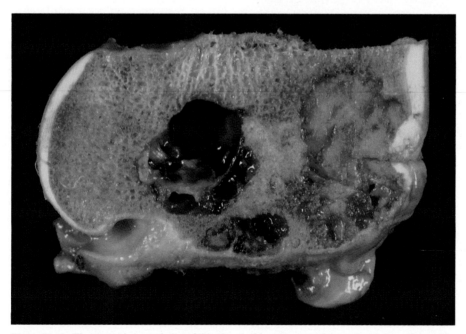

**Figure 11–2.** The gross characteristics of this chondroblastoma correlate well with its radiographic appearance in Figure 11–1. The lesion is fleshy and whitish in color in its solid regions. A hemorrhagic cystic region is also grossly evident. Secondary aneurysmal bone cyst quite frequently accompanies chondroblastoma.

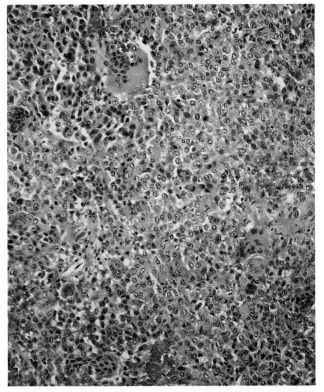

**Figure 11–3.** Chondroblastoma was originally thought to be a "calcifying giant cell tumor." The solid portion of the lesion may show numerous benign, multinucleated giant cells, as is illustrated in this photomicrograph.

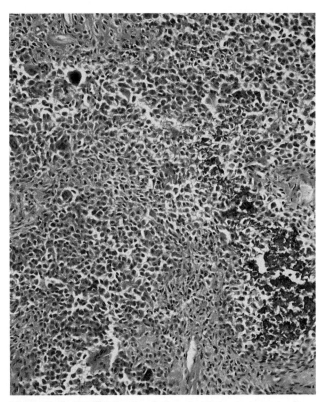

**Figure 11–5.** Calcification is a feature that helps to separate chondroblastoma from giant cell tumor. The calcification may be regional and identifiable radiographically, as is shown in this tumor. At times the calcification forms a "chicken wire"-type appearance.

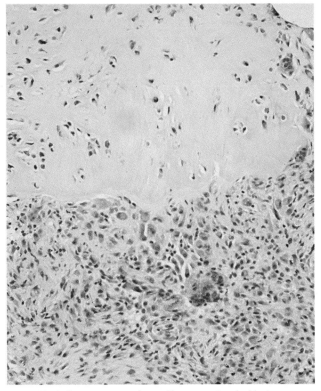

**Figure 11–4.** In contrast to giant cell tumor, chondroblastoma contains zones of eosinophilic to amphophilic fibrochondroid matrix, as is shown in this photomicrograph. These zones are typically hypocellular when compared with the surrounding regions.

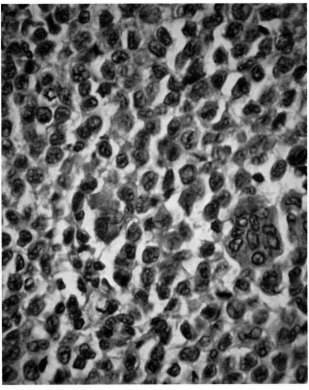

**Figure 11–6.** At high magnification chondroblastoma is generally loosely organized, as is shown in this photomicrograph. The nuclei are uniform and characteristically bean-shaped, with a central groove. This feature is similar to the cytologic appearance of the nuclei of Langerhans' cells of histiocytosis X.

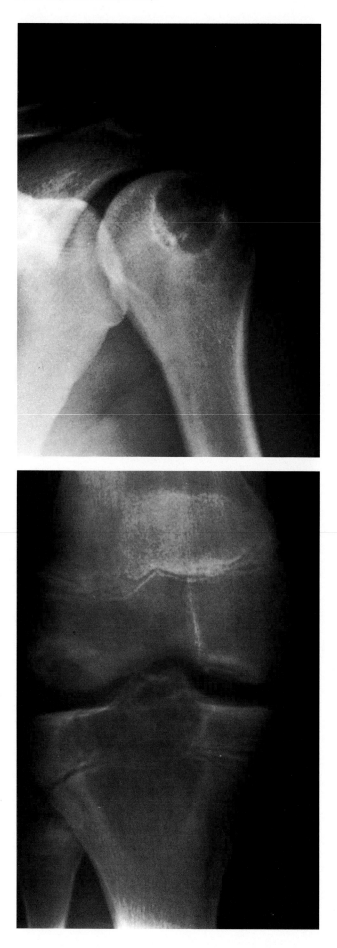

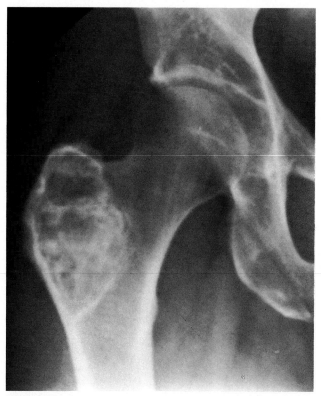

**Figure 11–7.** This radiograph illustrates a chondroblastoma involving the humeral head. In this region the lesion may involve the epiphysis or apophysis. Chondroblastomas are characteristically lytic, but this tumor shows partial calcification. A thin rim of sclerosis at the periphery attests to the lesion's slow growth.

**Figure 11–9.** Chondroblastomas show mineralization to varying degrees. This example involving the greater trochanter (apophyseal location) is heavily mineralized.

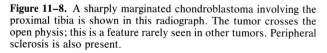

**Figure 11–8.** A sharply marginated chondroblastoma involving the proximal tibia is shown in this radiograph. The tumor crosses the open physis; this is a feature rarely seen in other tumors. Peripheral sclerosis is also present.

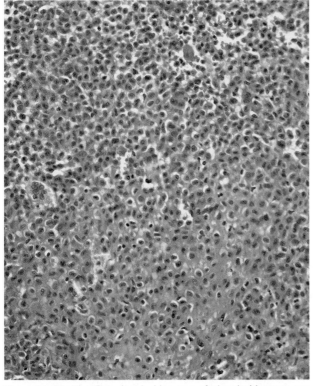

**Figure 11-10.** The fibrochondroid zones of chondroblastoma are variably scattered through the tumor and may not be a prominent component of the lesion, as in this case.

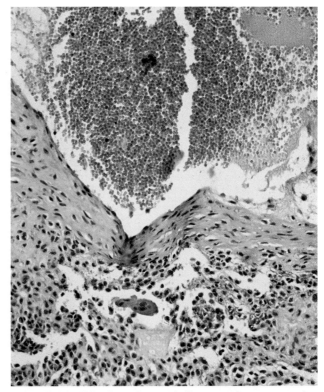

**Figure 11-12.** This photomicrograph illustrates the presence of a secondary aneurysmal bone cyst complicating a chondroblastoma. Such a secondary aneurysmal bone cyst may be so prominent as to mask the appearance of the chondroblastoma component and lead to a misdiagnosis.

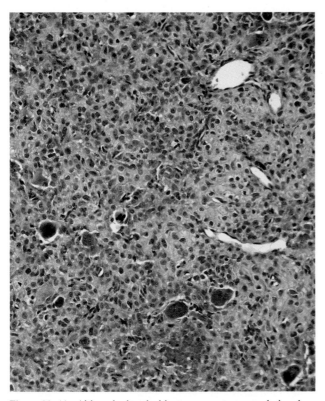

**Figure 11-11.** Although chondroblastoma most commonly involves the epiphyseal region of a long bone in a skeletally immature patient, some tumors occur in flat bones as well. This tumor involved the temporal bone in a three-year-old female. The temporal bone is the most common location for lesions involving the skull.

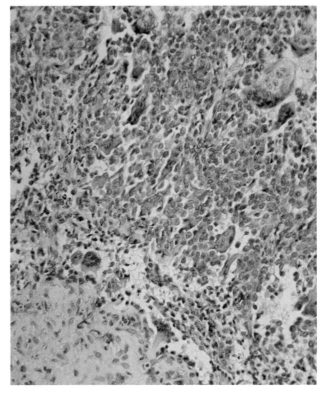

**Figure 11-13.** Chondroblastomas may recur within bone and soft tissue, and rarely such lesions may metastasize to the lungs. As this photomicrograph illustrates, such rare pulmonary metastases are histologically indistinguishable from their osseous primary lesions.

# CHAPTER 12

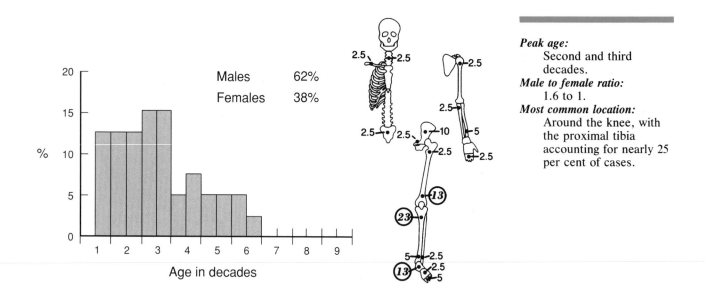

# Chondromyxoid Fibroma

Males 62%
Females 38%

% — Age in decades (chart, y-axis 0–20)

**Peak age:**
Second and third
decades.
**Male to female ratio:**
1.6 to 1.
**Most common location:**
Around the knee, with
the proximal tibia
accounting for nearly 25
per cent of cases.

■ **Clinical Symptoms**

1. Pain is the most common presenting complaint.
2. Local swelling may be noted on rare occasions
   and is more frequently a presenting complaint
   when the tumor involves a small bone.
3. Occasionally the lesion may be an asymptomatic, incidental radiographic abnormality.

■ **Clinical Signs**

1. Regional tenderness is usually the only finding
   on physical examination.
2. Tumefaction, as noted above, is more commonly
   found when the tumor involves bones of the
   hands or feet.

■ **Major Radiographic Features**

1. The lesion has an eccentric metaphyseal location.

2. It shows sharp, sclerotic, and scalloped margins.
3. Matrix calcification is rare.

■ **Radiographic Differential Diagnosis**

1. Fibroma (metaphyseal fibrous defect).
2. Aneurysmal bone cyst.
3. Chondroblastoma.
4. Fibrous dysplasia.

■ **Pathologic Features**

*Gross*

1. This tumor may grossly resemble hyaline cartilage, being translucent and bluish-gray in color;
   however, it is not soft and "runny" as in myxoid
   areas of chondrosarcoma.
2. The tumor is usually very well marginated and
   therefore may be lobulated grossly.
3. Bone surrounding the tumor usually shows sclerotic changes.

*Microscopic*

1. With low magnification the tumor shows a distinctly lobulated pattern of growth, with peripheral hypercellularity of the lobules.
2. The tumor cells are spindled and stellate in shape. Rarely the nuclei may appear "bizarre." Benign giant cells are usually seen between the lobules of the tumor.
3. The stroma is myxoid, but only rarely is well-formed hyaline cartilage seen.
4. More solidly cellular areas with cells identical with those seen in chondroblastoma may be seen.

■ **Pathologic Differential Diagnosis**

Benign lesions:
1. Chondroblastoma.
2. Chondroma.
Malignant lesions:
1. Chondrosarcoma.
2. Chondroblastic osteosarcoma.

■ **Treatment**

**Primary Modality:**   curettage and bone grafting.
**Other Possible Approaches:**   en bloc resection with a marginal margin if the tumor's location makes it amenable to removal without significant loss of function.

**References**

Gherlinzoni F, Rock M, and Picci P: Chondromyxoid fibroma: the experience at the Istituto Ortopedico Rizzoli. J Bone Joint Surg *65A*:198–204, 1983.

Kyriakos M: Soft tissue implantation of chondromyxoid fibroma. Am J Surg Pathol *3*:363–372, 1979.

Rahimi A, Beabout JW, Ivins JC, and Dahlin DC: Chondromyxoid fibroma: a clinicopathologic study of 76 cases. Cancer *30*:726–736, 1972.

Schajowicz F, and Gallardo J: Chondromyxoid fibroma (fibromyxoid chondroma) of bone: a clinicopathological study of thirty-two cases. J Bone Joint Surg *53B*:198–216, 1971.

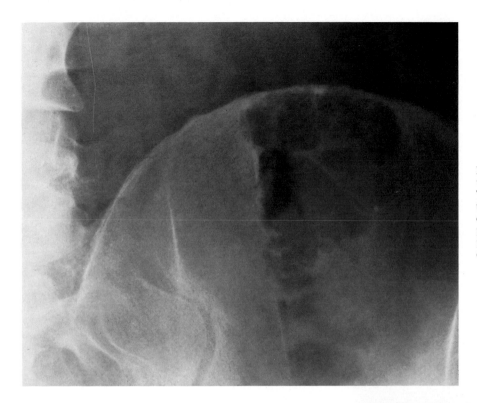

**Figure 12–1.** This radiograph shows a well-marginated lesion in the iliac bone. The periphery is scalloped and has a partially sclerotic rim. Although the majority of chondromyxoid fibromas are metaphyseal in long bones, approximately 10 per cent occur in the ilium (as in this case).

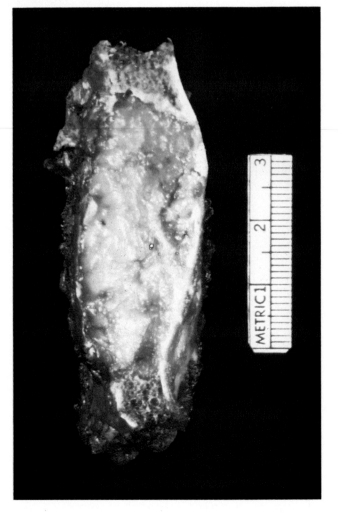

**Figure 12–2.** The gross features in this case correlate well with the radiograph shown in Figure 12–1. The lesion is whitish and well marginated. The lesion may show myxoid change.

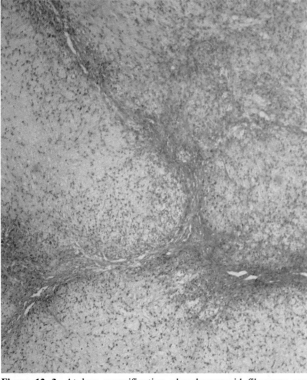

**Figure 12–3.** At low magnification chondromyxoid fibromas are characteristically lobulated, as this photomicrograph illustrates. The lesion is relatively hypocellular toward the center of the lobules.

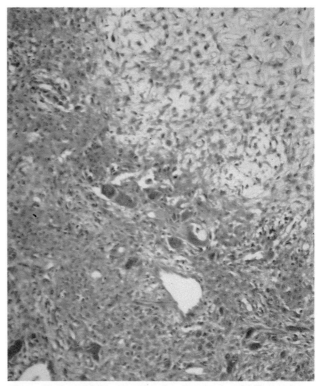

**Figure 12–5.** At higher magnification chondromyxoid fibroma has a chondroid appearance in the central portion of the tumor lobules. A small sampling of this portion of the lesional tissue may mimic the appearance of a chondroma or chondrosarcoma.

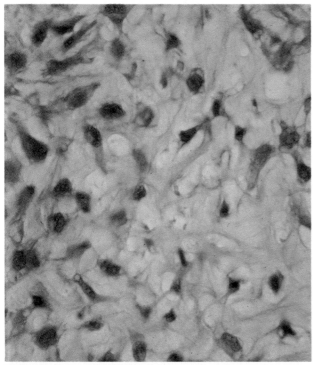

**Figure 12–4.** At the periphery of the lobules of tumor is a "condensation" of cellularity. In these regions the tumor tends to show more spindling, and benign multinucleated giant cells are present. These foci may mimic the appearance of chondroblastoma.

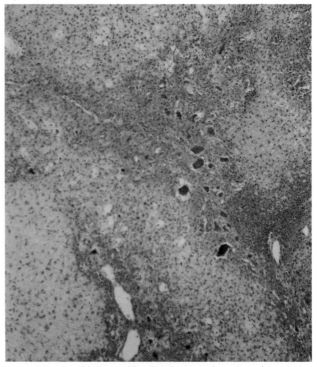

**Figure 12–6.** At high magnification the central portion of the tumor is chondromyxoid (well-developed hyaline cartilage is unusual in chondromyxoid fibroma). Cytologically the cells are stellate in shape in these regions. However, the nuclei are uniform and do not show significant atypia. Longitudinal grooves and a bean shape to the nucleus may simulate the cytologic features seen in chondroblastoma or histiocytosis X.

**Figure 12–8.** The lobulated radiographic appearance of a chondro-myxoid fibroma is demonstrated in this case. The differential diagnosis in such a case would include a metaphyseal fibrous defect (fibroma).

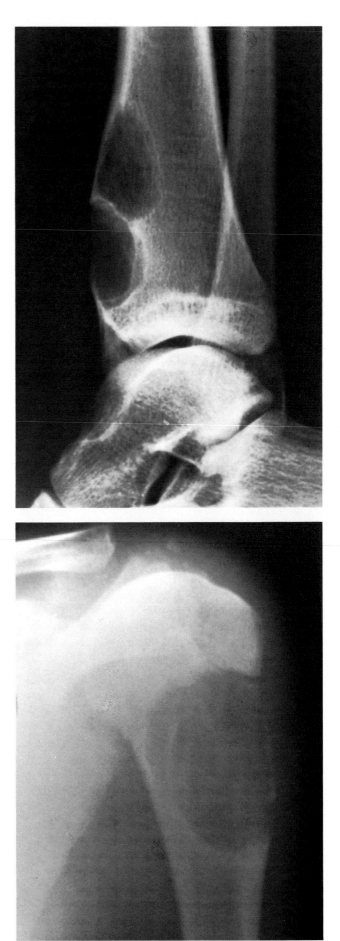

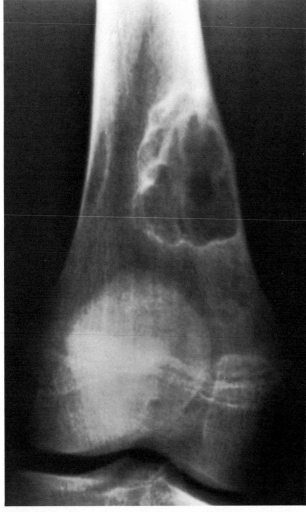

**Figure 12–7.** This radiograph illustrates the features of a chondro-myxoid fibroma in the distal femur. The metaphyseal location is typical, and the lesion is eccentric. The sclerotic and scalloped rim is clearly visible in this case.

**Figure 12–9.** This chondromyxoid fibroma of the upper humerus again shows a lytic and well-marginated radiographic appearance. The lesion abuts but does not cross the physis.

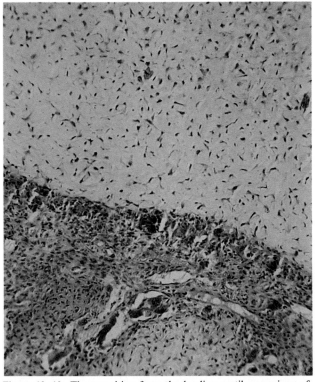

**Figure 12–10.** The transition from the hyaline cartilage regions of the tumor to the more cellular areas may be quite abrupt, as is shown in this photomicrograph. The tumor may thus exhibit a "bimorphic" histologic pattern.

**Figure 12–12.** Foci within a chondromyxoid fibroma may be markedly chondroid and thus simulate a chondroma or chondrosarcoma. Chondromyxoid fibromas were commonly mistaken for chondrosarcomas in the past, but the publication of this fact has resulted in more mistaken identifications of chondrosarcomas as chondromyxoid fibromas in recent years.

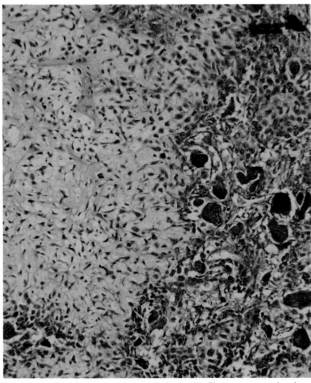

**Figure 12–11.** Regions of chondromyxoid fibroma may simulate chondroblastoma, as this photomicrograph illustrates. The cytologic features also overlap, suggesting that the two lesions are closely related.

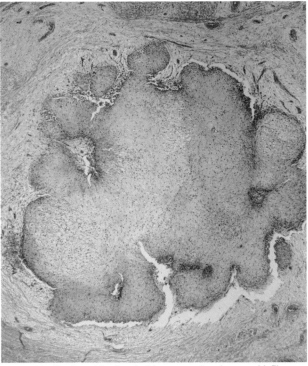

**Figure 12–13.** As with chondroblastoma, chondromyxoid fibroma may recur if inadequately treated. The recurrence may be within the bone or soft tissues, as is shown in this photomicrograph. Such soft tissue recurrences frequently show a rim of calcification radiographically.

# CHAPTER 13

## Multiple Chondromas

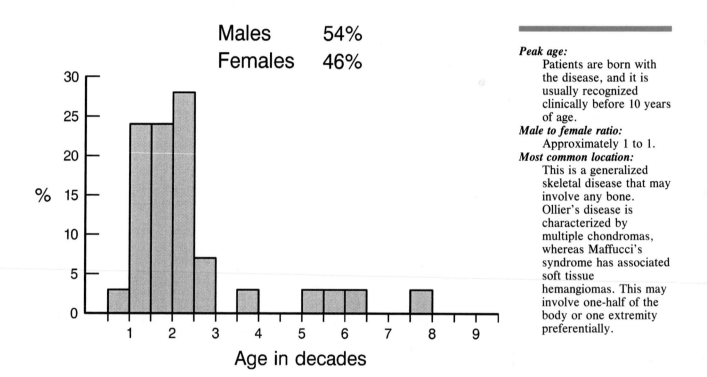

Males      54%
Females    46%

% / Age in decades

*Peak age:*
Patients are born with the disease, and it is usually recognized clinically before 10 years of age.

*Male to female ratio:*
Approximately 1 to 1.

*Most common location:*
This is a generalized skeletal disease that may involve any bone. Ollier's disease is characterized by multiple chondromas, whereas Maffucci's syndrome has associated soft tissue hemangiomas. This may involve one-half of the body or one extremity preferentially.

■ **Clinical Symptoms**

1. Symptoms are similar to those of the solitary lesion, with pain and associated pathologic fracture.

■ **Clinical Signs**

1. Multiple mass lesions are palpable.
2. Deformity and shortness of stature are often present because of epiphyseal involvement.
3. There is a tendency to unilaterality in Ollier's disease.
4. Hemangiomas are associated with Maffucci's syndrome.

■ **Major Radiographic Features**

1. Most cases are bilateral, but involvement usually predominates on one side.
2. Affected bones are shortened and deformed.
3. Cartilage masses extend linearly from the physis into the metaphysis.
4. Cartilage masses often have no overlying cortex and may contain stippled calcification.
5. There is a tendency to spare the epiphysis and diaphysis except in severe cases.
6. Affected bones cannot tubulate, and the ends may have a clubbed appearance.
7. The disease tends to regress after puberty.

■ **Radiographic Differential Diagnosis**

1. Fibrous dysplasia.
2. Multiple hereditary exostoses.

■ **Pathologic Features**

*Gross*

1. The lesional tissue is blue-gray and translucent in appearance.
2. No myxoid or cystic change is evident grossly.

*Microscopic*

1. On low magnification these lesions are composed predominantly of blue-gray hyaline cartilage matrix.
2. The lesions are generally more cellular than is seen in solitary chondromas. No myxoid stromal change is evident.
3. On higher magnification, the nuclei may be hyperchromic and binucleated cells may be identified.

■ **Pathologic Differential Diagnosis**

Benign lesions:
1. Solitary chondroma.
2. Synovial chondromatosis.
Malignant lesions:
1. Chondrosarcoma, ordinary type.

■ **Treatment**

**Primary Modality:** Treatment is similar to that for solitary enchondromas, with observation of the lesions if they are asymptomatic.
**Other Possible Approaches:** curettage and bone grafting of the lesion if it is symptomatic.

### References

Loewinger RJ, Lichtenstein JR, Dodson WE, et al: Maffucci's syndrome: amesenchymal dysplasia and multiple tumour syndrome. Br. J. Dermatol. *96*:317–322, 1977.
Nardell SG: Ollier's disease: dyschondroplasia. Br. Med. J. *2*:555–557, 1950.

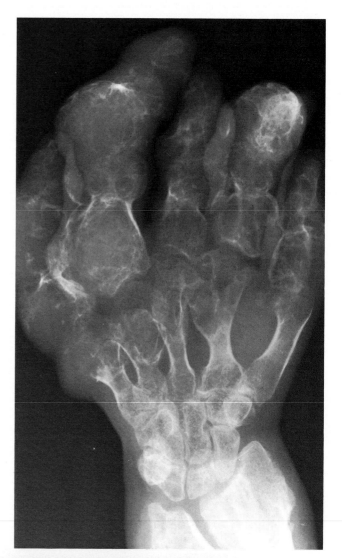

**Figure 13–1.** This radiograph illustrates extreme deformity of the bones of the hand and wrist by numerous masses of cartilage.

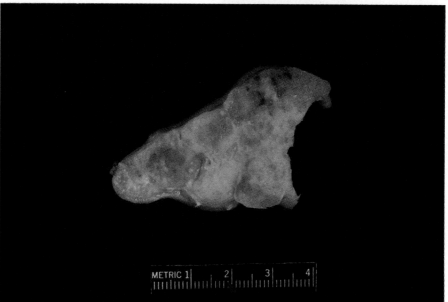

**Figure 13–2.** This gross photograph illustrates the features of multiple chondromas in Ollier's disease involving the fifth finger. The disease had resulted in such bony deformity that amputation was done.

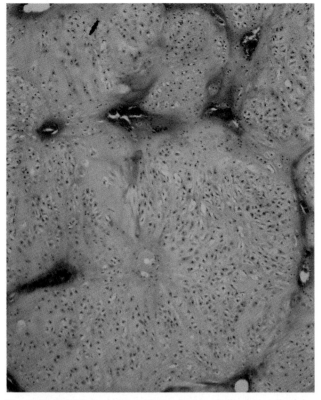

**Figure 13–3.** This low-power photomicrograph illustrates the lobulated appearance of a chondroma in Ollier's disease. This lesion of the humerus shows somewhat greater cellularity than is seen in many solitary chondromas of the long bones.

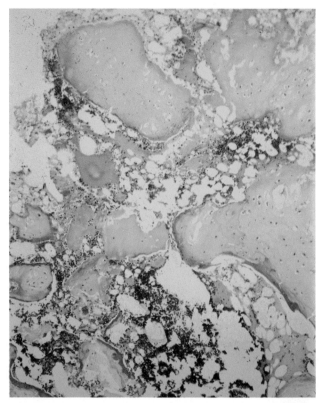

**Figure 13–5.** The multifocal nature of the chondromas in Ollier's disease is sometimes appreciable histologically, as in this example.

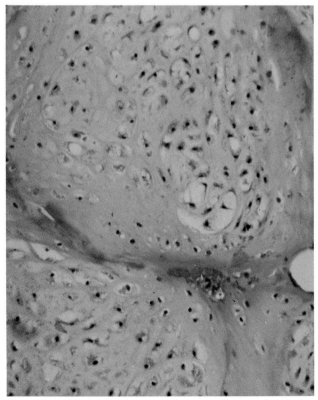

**Figure 13–4.** The lobulated nature of the chondromas in Ollier's disease is shown at higher magnification in this photomicrograph. Some mild cytologic atypia is also evident in this humeral lesion.

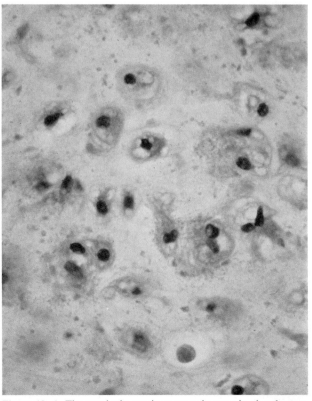

**Figure 13–6.** The cytologic atypia commonly seen in chondromas of the small bones of the hands and feet can also be seen in Ollier's disease, as is demonstrated in this lesion of the thumb.

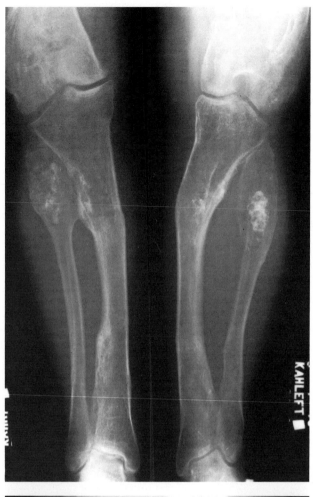

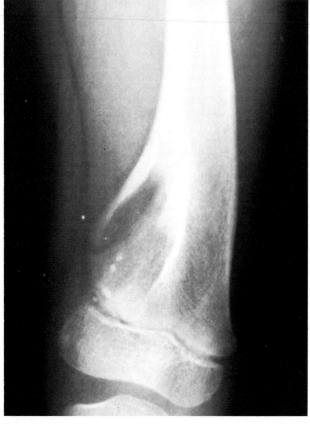

**Figure 13–7.** Ollier's disease of the lower legs with bowing, expansion, and deformity of the tibia and fibula is illustrated in this radiograph. Multiple cartilage masses containing stippled calcification are evident.

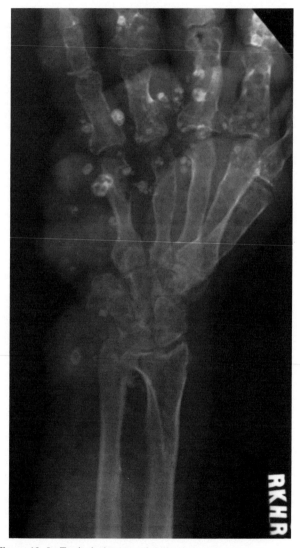

**Figure 13–9.** Typical changes of Ollier's disease in the bones associated with soft tissue hemangiomas containing phleboliths are shown in this example of Maffucci's syndrome.

**Figure 13–8.** Cartilage mass extending linearly from the physis into the metaphysis is noted in this example of Ollier's disease in a four-year-old male patient. There is absence of overlying cortex, and stippled calcification is present.

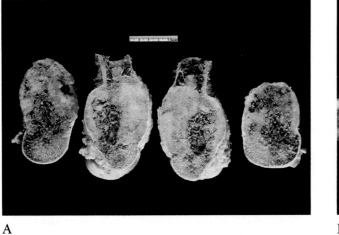

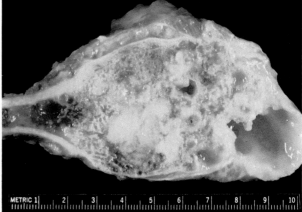

A                                                    B

**Figure 13–10.** Chondrosarcomas can be seen in association with the multiple chondroma syndromes of Ollier's disease (distal femoral tumor shown in *A*) and Maffucci's syndrome (proximal fibular chondrosarcoma shown in *B*).

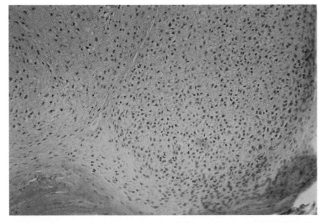

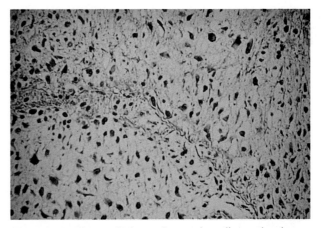

**Figure 13–11.** Chondrosarcomas in Ollier's disease and Maffucci's syndrome show the cellularity typical of low-grade chondrosarcomas not associated with multiple chondroma syndromes. This Grade 1 chondrosarcoma is from the proximal ulna in a patient with Ollier's disease.

**Figure 13–12.** The cytologic atypia seen in ordinary chondrosarcomas is also evident in chondrosarcomas complicating Ollier's disease, as is illustrated in this case involving the tibia.

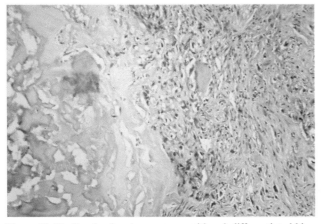

**Figure 13–13.** Rarely chondrosarcomas with a dedifferentiated histologic appearance have been identified arising in the background of Ollier's disease, as is shown in this case involving the femur.

# CHAPTER 14

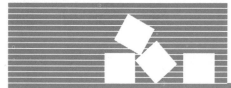

# Periosteal Chondroma

Males 65%
Females 35%

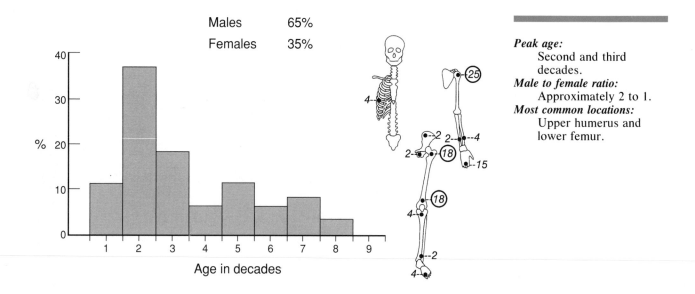

% (y-axis) 0, 10, 20, 30, 40

Age in decades (x-axis) 1–9

**Peak age:**
Second and third decades.
**Male to female ratio:**
Approximately 2 to 1.
**Most common locations:**
Upper humerus and lower femur.

■ **Clinical Symptoms**

1. Patients usually are asymptomatic.
2. The lesion is most commonly an incidental finding on radiographic examination.

■ **Clinical Signs**

1. The lesion may be palpable on physical examination.
2. The lesion is usually not painful to palpation.

■ **Major Radiographic Features**

1. The lesion consists of a small surface mass (less than 3 cm) with saucerization of the underlying bone.
2. It is metaphyseal or diaphyseal in location.
3. Marginal spicules or "buttresses" are present.
4. Approximately 33 per cent are calcified.

■ **Radiographic Differential Diagnosis**

1. Periosteal chondrosarcoma.
2. Periosteal osteosarcoma.
3. Soft tissue neoplasm secondarily involving the cortical bone.

■ **Pathologic Features**

*Gross*

1. The tumor is gray-blue and translucent, like all tumors with a prominent hyaline cartilage component.
2. If the margin is present in the specimen, it shows sharp circumscription.
3. The medullary portion of the bone is not involved.
4. The tumor is firm and lacks liquefaction or cystic change.

*Microscopic*

1. The low-power histologic appearance is that of a lobulated hyaline cartilage tumor that is well circumscribed.
2. The lesion is usually hypercellular.
3. The lesion usually contains binucleated chondrocytes.
4. Nuclear atypia may be prominent.

## ■ Pathologic Differential Diagnosis

Benign lesions:
1. Synovial chondromatosis.
2. Chondroma.

Malignant lesions:
1. Periosteal chondrosarcoma.
2. Periosteal osteosarcoma.

## ■ Treatment

**Primary Modality:**  These lesions should be excised en bloc with a marginal or wide margin. Depending on the size of the defect, bone grafting may be necessary.

**Other Possible Approaches:**  observation, if a diagnosis is secure and the patient is asymptomatic.

## References

Bauer TW, Dorfman HD, and Latham JT Jr: Periosteal chondroma: a clinicopathologic study of 23 cases. Am J Surg Pathol 6:631–637, 1982.

Boriani S, Bacchini P, Bertoni F, and Campanacci M: Periosteal chondroma: a review of twenty cases. J Bone Joint Surg 65A:205–212, 1983.

DeSantos LA, and Spjut JH: Periosteal chondroma: a radiographic spectrum. Skeletal Radiol 6:15–20, 1981.

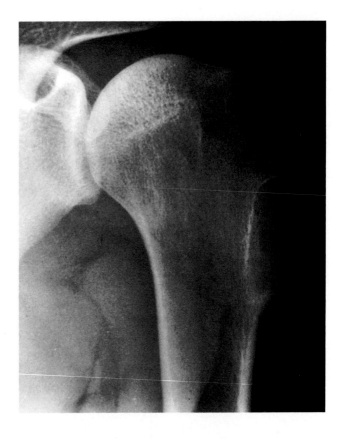

**Figure 14–1.** This radiograph shows a small periosteal chondroma arising on the lateral surface of the upper humeral metaphysis. The sharp margination and thin sclerotic rim, as well as the marginal spicules of calcification, are typical of periosteal chondroma. An incomplete rim of calcification surrounds the soft tissue component of this lesion.

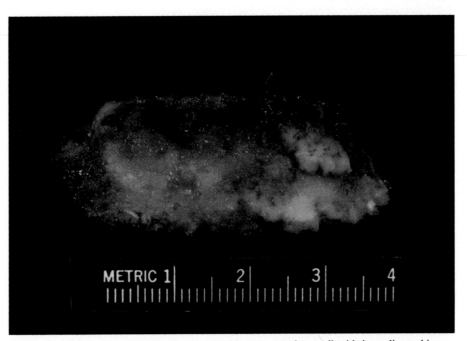

**Figure 14–2.** The gross pathologic features in this case correlate well with its radiographic appearance in Figure 14–1. The small size of the lesion supports a benign diagnosis. As with other hyaline cartilage lesions, the tumor is blue-gray in color and glistening.

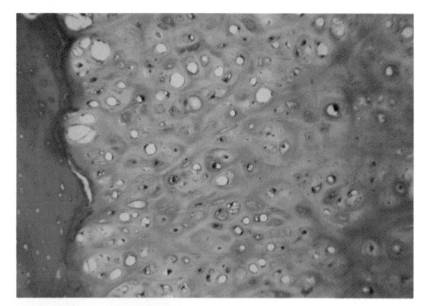

**Figure 14–3.** At low magnification a periosteal chondroma is hypocellular and well circumscribed. This photomicrograph shows that the tumor has not penetrated the underlying cortical bone.

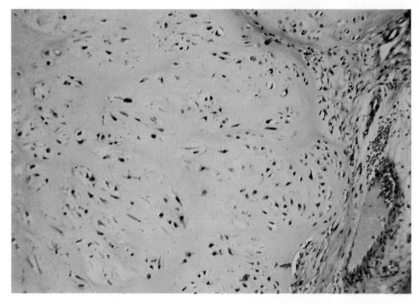

**Figure 14–4.** The lobulated pattern of a hyaline cartilage tumor is shown in this photomicrograph. Although periosteal chondromas are benign, they may show greater cellularity at low magnification than their intramedullary counterparts.

**Figure 14–5.** At high magnification the cytologic features of the chondrocytes are uniform. Binucleation, as is seen in this photomicrograph, should not dissuade the pathologist from making a diagnosis of periosteal chondroma if the gross and radiographic features are typical.

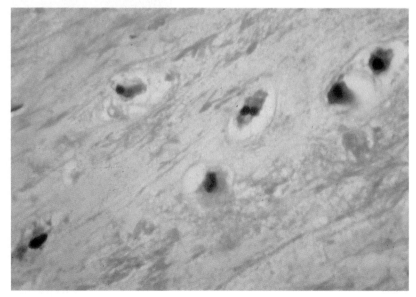

**Figure 14–7.** Mineralization need not be present in periosteal chondromas, as is shown by this example of a distal femoral lesion, which otherwise exhibits typical radiographic features of periosteal chondroma.

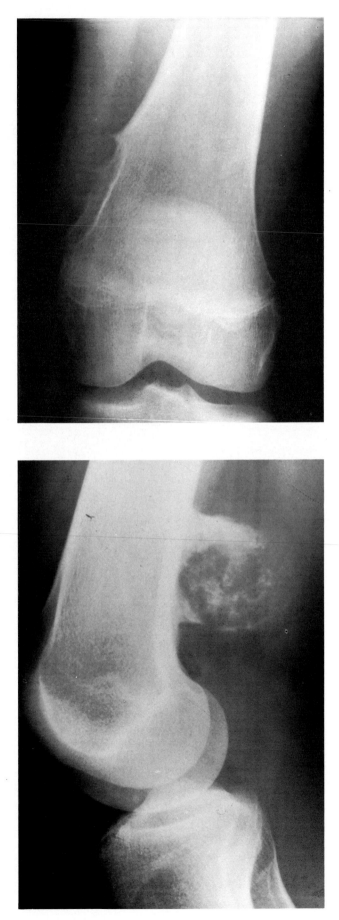

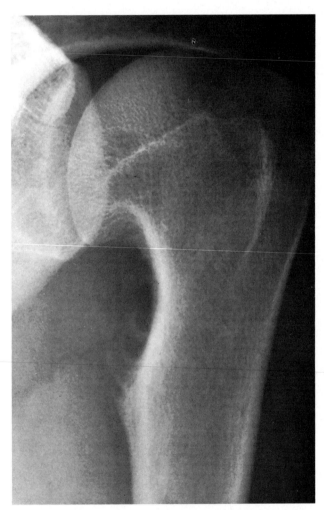

**Figure 14–6.** This radiograph illustrates a periosteal chondroma of the proximal humerus. The lesion shows a sharp sclerotic margin indicative of slow growth. The marginal spicules and buttresses are typical of periosteal chondroma.

**Figure 14–8.** This partially calcified periosteal chondroma of the posterior distal femur occupies the most common location of a parosteal osteosarcoma. However, the mineralization present is typical of a hyaline cartilage lesion. As such, periosteal osteosarcoma is more frequently in the radiographic differential diagnosis with periosteal chondroma.

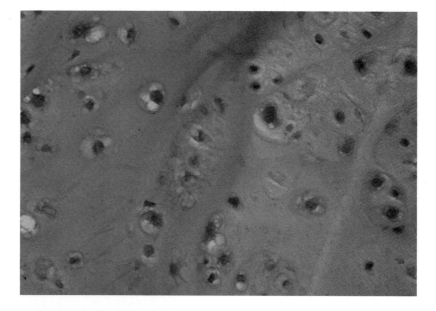

**Figure 14–9.** At high magnification, periosteal chondromas frequently show greater nuclear pleomorphism and more numerous binucleation than intramedullary chondromas. Thus the histologic features of periosteal chondroma are closer to chondromas of the small bones and synovial chondromatosis.

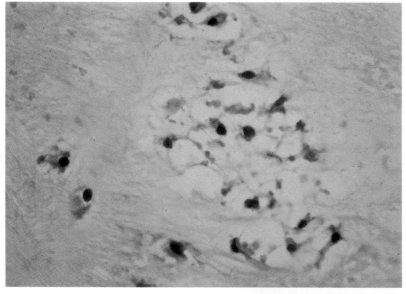

**Figure 14–10.** Focal myxoid change may be seen in a periosteal chondroma, as is illustrated in this photomicrograph. Such a feature, however, should alert the pathologist to carefully evaluate the lesion.

**Figure 14–11.** This gross specimen shows a periosteal chondrosarcoma. In contrast to periosteal chondromas, which are 3 cm or less in size, periosteal chondrosarcomas are 5 cm or larger, as is shown in this photograph of a femoral lesion.

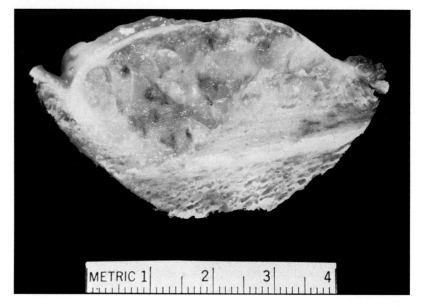

# CHAPTER 15

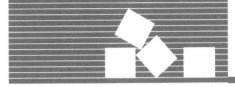

# Chondrosarcoma

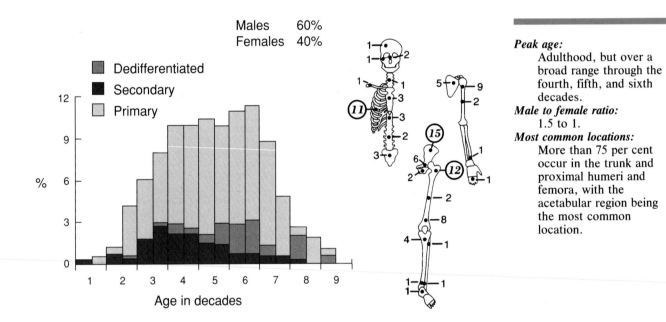

Males 60%
Females 40%

- Dedifferentiated
- Secondary
- Primary

*Peak age:*
   Adulthood, but over a broad range through the fourth, fifth, and sixth decades.
*Male to female ratio:*
   1.5 to 1.
*Most common locations:*
   More than 75 per cent occur in the trunk and proximal humeri and femora, with the acetabular region being the most common location.

## ■ Clinical Symptoms

1. Pain is the usual presenting complaint. The pain is usually local; however, when tumors involve the pelvic girdle or vertebra, referred pain may be the initial manifestation.
2. A mass lesion may be noted but is more commonly present in patients who have tumors involving the appendicular skeleton.
3. A long duration of clinical symptoms—even of one or two decades—is frequently seen, since these tumors almost invariably are slow growing.

## ■ Clinical Signs

1. Local tenderness is present.
2. A mass may be found on physical examination. The mass is generally hard.

## ■ Major Radiographic Features

1. There is a predilection for the central skeleton and for the metaphysis or diaphysis of the affected bone.
2. Sixty-six per cent of lesions are partially calcified.
3. Cortical erosion or destruction is usually present.
4. The cortex is often thickened, but periosteal reaction is scant or absent.
5. Soft tissue extension is commonly seen in large lesions.

## ■ Radiographic Differential Diagnosis

1. Osteosarcoma.
2. Fibrosarcoma.

3. Metastatic carcinoma.
4. Multiple myeloma.

## ■ Pathologic Features

### Gross

1. Chondrosarcomas tend to be homogeneous and blue-gray in color.
2. Scattered regions of whitish-yellow calcification may be evident.
3. Myxoid foci or frank liquefaction of the tumor helps to grossly separate chondrosarcoma from chondroma.

### Microscopic

1. With low magnification these tumors show abundant blue-gray chondroid matrix production.
2. The tumors vary in cellularity but in general are more cellular than chondromas. The grade of the tumor correlates in general with its cellularity; higher-grade tumors are more cellular.
3. On higher magnification, the nuclei of the cells are somewhat variable and are more pleomorphic than the cells of a chondroma.
4. Binucleation of the cells is frequently evident but is not a feature that suffices for a diagnosis of malignancy, since some chondromas also show this feature.
5. Myxoid change within the chondroid matrix may be evidenced by an inhomogeneous and "stringy" appearance. This is a particularly important histologic feature to help separate chondroma from low-grade chondrosarcoma in long bones.
6. The cytologic atypia evident on high-power examination is generally mild to moderate. If a tumor with marked cytologic atypia is encountered, a careful search should be made for osteoid production to exclude the diagnosis of chondroblastic osteosarcoma.
7. The guidelines for a diagnosis of chondrosarcoma in a small bone of the hand or foot are different. Increased cellularity, binucleated cells, hyperchromasia, and myxoid change may

all be present in a chondroma in this location. Radiologic evidence of permeation of the tumor through the cortex should be present in order to diagnose chondrosarcoma in these locations.

## ■ Pathologic Differential Diagnosis

Benign lesions:
1. Chondroma.
2. Chondromyxoid fibroma.
Malignant lesions:
1. Chondroblastic osteosarcoma.
2. Chondroid chordoma.

## ■ Treatment

**Primary Modality:** surgical resection with a wide surgical margin. Reconstruction is individualized depending on the location of the lesion. Amputation may be necessary to achieve a wide surgical margin.

**Other Possible Approaches:** Although these tumors are considered to be resistant to routine chemotherapy and radiation therapy, radiation is used for palliation in surgically inaccessible sites such as the spine or sacrum.

## References

Bjornsson J, Unni KK, Dahlin DC, et al: Clear cell chondrosarcoma of bone: observations in 47 cases. Am J Surg Pathol 8:223–230, 1984.

Faraggiana T, Sendser B, and Glicksman LP: Light- and electron-microscopic study of clear cell chondrosarcoma. Am J Clin Pathol 75:117–121, 1981.

Garrison RC, Unni KK, McLeod RA, et al: Chondrosarcoma arising in osteochondroma. Cancer 49:1890–1897, 1982.

Gitelis S, Bertoni F, Picci P, and Campanacci M: Chondrosarcoma of bone: the experience at the Istituto Ortopedico Rizzoli. J Bone Joint Surg 63A:1248–1257, 1981.

Mankin JH, Cantley KP, Lippiello L, et al: The biology of human chondrosarcoma. I. Description of the cases, grading, and biochemical analyses. J Bone Joint Surg 62A:160–176, 1980.

McCarthy EF, and Dorfman HD: Chondrosarcoma of bone with dedifferentiation: a study of eighteen cases. Hum Pathol 13:36–40, 1982.

Pritchard DJ, Lunke RJ, Taylor WF, et al: Chondrosarcoma: a clinicopathologic and statistical analysis. Cancer 45:149–157, 1980.

Rosenthal DI, Schiller AL, and Mankin JH: Chondrosarcoma: correlation of radiological and histological grade. Radiology 150:21–26, 1984.

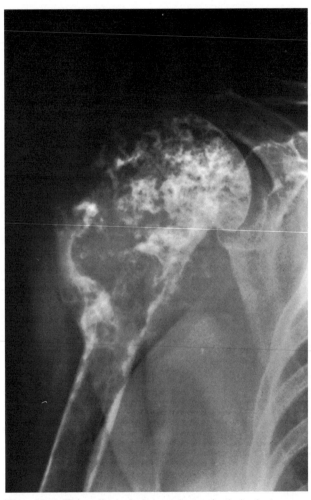

**Figure 15–1.** This radiograph shows a destructive lesion in the proximal humerus in an adult patient. The lesion is partially calcified, showing multiple areas of ring-like calcification. These features are indicative of a hyaline cartilage tumor. The extensive cortical destruction and associated soft tissue extension of the tumor support a malignant diagnosis.

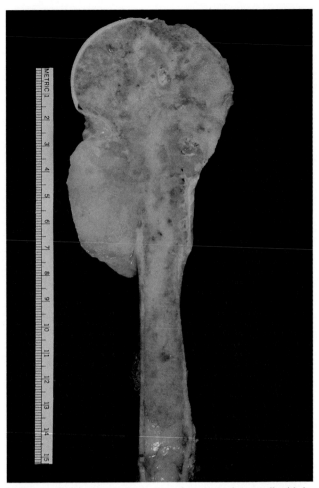

**Figure 15–2.** The bisected gross specimen correlates well with its radiographic appearance shown in Figure 15–1. The tumor shows the characteristic blue-gray aura of a hyaline cartilage tumor on cross-section. The cortex has been destroyed, and an associated soft tissue mass is present.

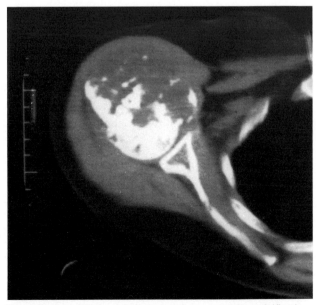

**Figure 15–3.** A CT scan of this lesion shows extensive calcification. CT and MRI are particularly helpful in defining the extent of soft tissue involvement and the relationship of any soft tissue extension to regional neurovascular structures.

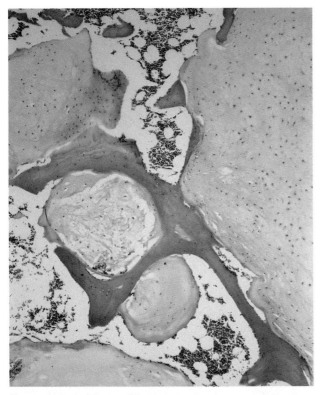

**Figure 15–4.** At low magnification chondrosarcomas are blue-gray with hematoxylin- and eosin-stained sections. The tumors are generally not highly cellular but are often arranged in a lobulated manner. Adjacent lobules at the periphery of the lesion show an invasive quality of growth, as is illustrated in this photomicrograph.

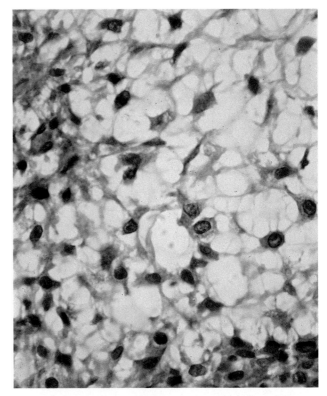

**Figure 15–6.** At higher magnification the nuclear pleomorphism is more evident. This tumor also shows a myxoid stromal quality, a feature that is frequently seen in chondrosarcomas.

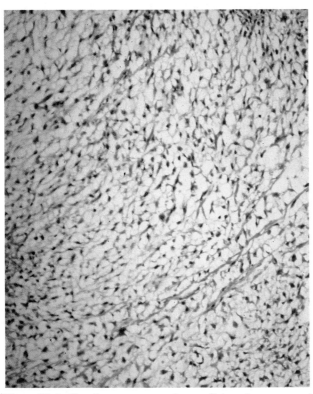

**Figure 15–5.** Chondrosarcomas are hypercellular when compared with chondromas, as is shown in this example of a chondrosarcoma of the distal femur. The nuclei show greater pleomorphism and are hyperchromatic as well.

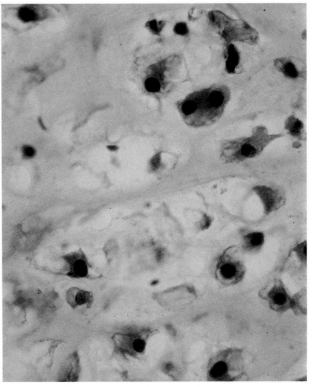

**Figure 15–7.** Binucleation is commonly stated to be an important feature in the differentiation of chondrosarcoma from chondroma. Binucleated chondrocytes are identifiable in this example of a chondrosarcoma involving the sacroiliac region.

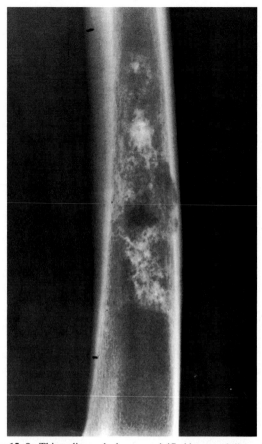

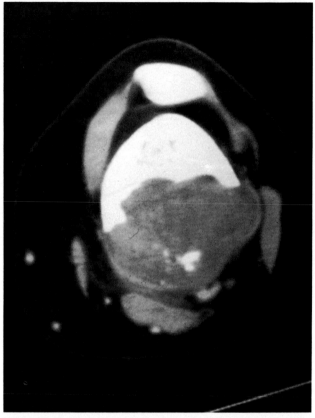

**Figure 15–8.** This radiograph shows a calcified intramedullary chondrosarcoma of the femoral diaphysis. Central lysis and cortical erosion are present and constitute the major radiographic evidence that the lesion is malignant.

**Figure 15–10.** Destruction of the cortex is associated with a bulky soft tissue mass in this case. An area of central calcification is also present. CT and MRI are essential modalities for preoperative staging. This CT scan demonstrates the extent of this chondrosarcoma and the presence of subtle calcification, which help identify the tumor as most probably being a chondrosarcoma.

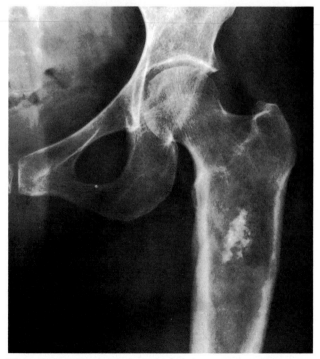

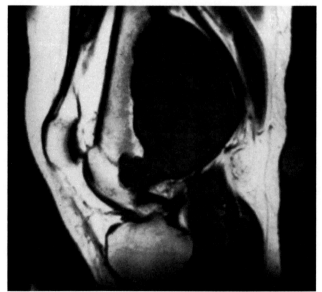

**Figure 15–9.** This chondrosarcoma is large, partially calcified, and poorly marginated. Expansion of the bone in combination with cortical thickening, as is seen in this case, is unusual in any tumor other than chondrosarcoma.

**Figure 15–11.** MRI provides superior contrast between the tumor and normal marrow as well as between the tumor and adjacent soft tissues, as is demonstrated in this image showing the same tumor seen in the CT scan in Figure 15–10. Sagittal images are useful in showing the longitudinal extent of the tumor in a single slice. Calcification is not demonstrated.

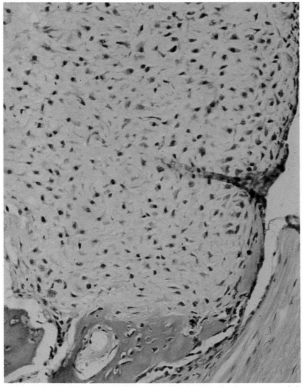

**Figure 15–12.** This photomicrograph illustrates the low-power, lobulated pattern of growth present in a chondrosarcoma.

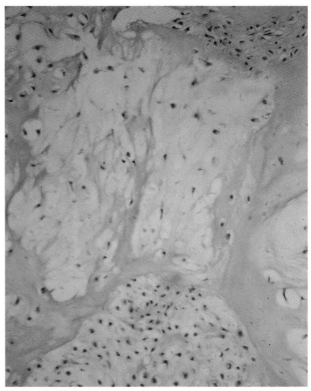

**Figure 15–14.** At low power, the myxoid quality of the lesion may be the first clue that the hyaline cartilage tumor is not a chondroma. This photomicrograph shows such a stromal myxoid change.

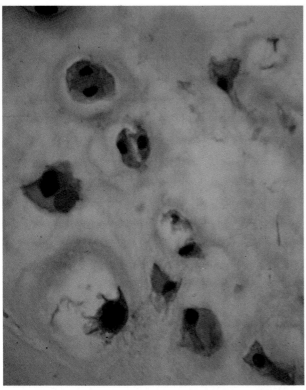

**Figure 15–13.** Multiple binucleated chondrocytes are identifiable in this high-power photomicrograph of a chondrosarcoma. Nuclear pleomorphism is also evident. Although chondromas of the small bones, periosteal chondromas, and synovial chondromatosis may also share these features, they are not present to the extent illustrated here.

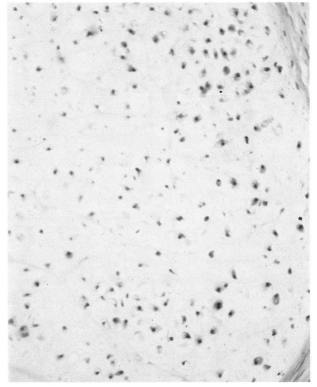

**Figure 15–15.** As the majority of chondrosarcomas are low-grade, the histologic features alone may not be sufficient to support a malignant diagnosis. Although slightly hypercellular, the location of the tumor (non–small bone and not periosteal) and the radiographic features showing endosteal erosion would be particularly helpful in classifying this tumor as malignant.

# CHAPTER 16

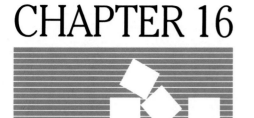

# Chondrosarcoma Arising in Osteochondroma

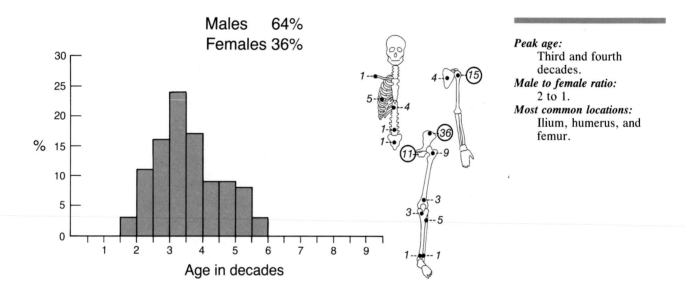

Males    64%
Females 36%

% (y-axis), Age in decades (x-axis)

**Peak age:**
Third and fourth
decades.
**Male to female ratio:**
2 to 1.
**Most common locations:**
Ilium, humerus, and
femur.

■ **Clinical Symptoms**

1. A mass lesion that may have recently increased in size is found.
2. Pain is present in the region of the lesion.

■ **Clinical Signs**

1. A tender mass lesion is present.

■ **Major Radiographic Features**

1. A thick and indistinct cartilage cap may be seen on a lesion that otherwise has the features of an osteochondroma.
2. Radiolucent regions in the lesion are a useful indicator of secondary chondrosarcoma when present.

3. Destruction of the underlying osteochondroma or adjacent bone is evident in advanced cases.
4. MRI and computed tomography (CT) are the most sensitive diagnostic techniques for assessing these radiographic features.

■ **Radiographic Differential Diagnosis**

1. Osteochondroma with secondary bursa formation.
2. Atypical benign osteochondroma.

■ **Pathologic Features**

*Gross*

1. Masses of cartilaginous tissue greater than 2 cm in thickness are present.
2. The cartilaginous tissue may show liquefaction or frank cystification.

3. There is extension into the surrounding soft tissues.

### Microscopic

1. On low-power examination the tumor is composed predominantly of hyaline cartilage.
2. Most tumors are hypocellular but show greater cytologic atypia than is seen in an osteochondroma.
3. The cartilage cap is not arranged in the orderly columnar manner present in an osteochondroma but rather is disorganized, with clusters of cells scattered in the cartilage matrix.
4. Myxoid change characterized by a loose, watery appearance of the cartilage matrix or by a stringing of the matrix is evident.

### ■ Pathologic Differential Diagnosis

Benign lesions:

1. Osteochondroma.
2. Periosteal chondroma.

Malignant lesions:

1. Periosteal chondrosarcoma.
2. Periosteal osteosarcoma.

### ■ Treatment

**Primary Modality:** surgical resection with a wide margin. Bone grafting of the cortical defect is usually necessary. Other bone and joint reconstructive procedures may be indicated, depending on the size of the defect.

**Other Possible Approaches:** amputation, if a wide margin cannot be achieved by resection owing to soft tissue or neurovascular involvement.

### Reference

Garrison RC, Unni KK, McLeod RA, et al: Chondrosarcoma arising in osteochondroma. Cancer 49:1890–1897, 1982.

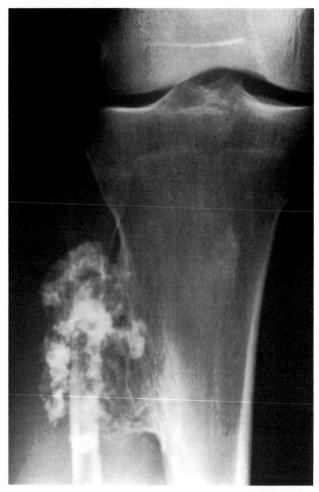

**Figure 16–1.** This radiograph illustrates a typical osteochondroma arising from the diametaphyseal region of the proximal tibia. The surface is indistinct and irregular, with some areas lacking calcification. These features suggest the possibility of a chondrosarcoma arising in the osteochondroma.

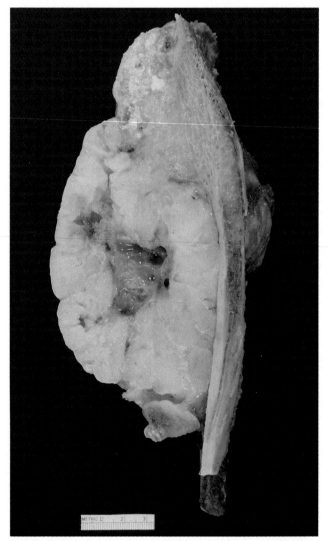

**Figure 16–2.** The gross pathologic features in this case mirror the radiographic appearance of the lesion. The thickness of the cartilage (more than 2 cm) indicates that the tumor may be malignant. In addition, the central portion of the hyaline cartilage tumor has undergone myxoid degeneration, a gross pathologic feature commonly associated with malignancy.

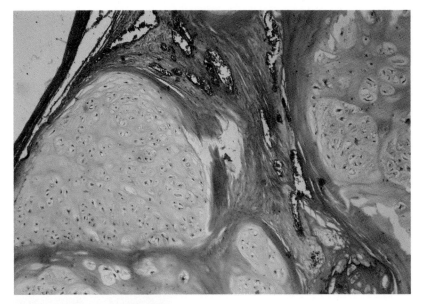

**Figure 16–3.** At low magnification, the periphery of a chondrosarcoma arising in an osteochondroma may show invasion, as is illustrated in this photomicrograph. The lobulated nature of the lesion is also evident at low power, and the tumor is more cellular than the cartilage cap of an osteochondroma.

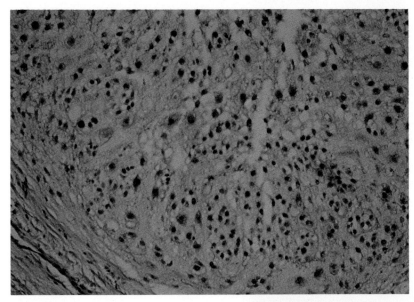

**Figure 16–4.** At higher magnification the cellularity of the lesion and the cytologic atypia are evident. The nuclear pleomorphism and cellularity are equivalent to that seen in intramedullary chondrosarcoma.

**Figure 16–5.** Invasion of the soft tissues adjacent to the lesion is helpful in identifying the tumor as malignant. However, bursa formation can occur in the region of an osteochondroma and radiographically mimic the appearance of soft tissue invasion.

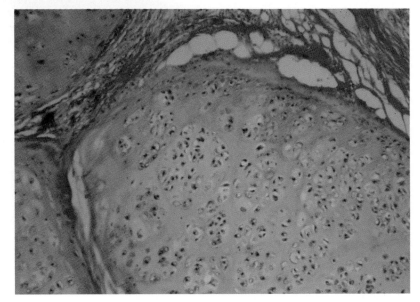

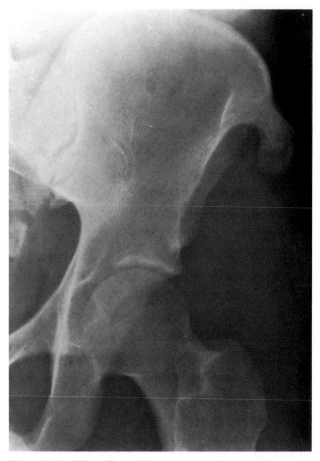

**Figure 16–6.** This radiograph demonstrates the typical features of an osteochondroma involving the iliac bone.

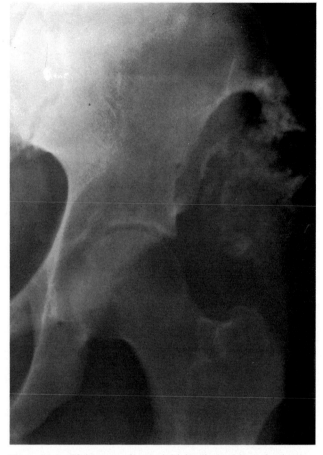

**Figure 16–7.** Eight years after the initial radiographic evaluation (see Fig. 16–6), the lesion is markedly enlarged and the periphery is indistinct. A secondary chondrosarcoma has developed in the lesion.

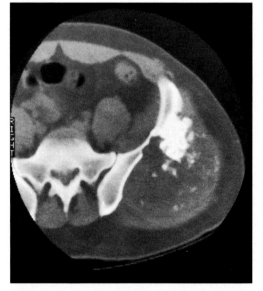

**Figure 16–8.** This CT scan shows a chondrosarcoma arising in an osteochondroma of the iliac bone. Soft tissue masses may be more easily evaluated with this imaging modality. Note that the soft tissue component of this lesion shows scanty calcification.

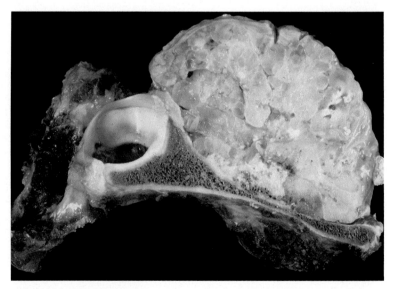

**Figure 16–9.** This gross specimen shows a secondary chondrosarcoma arising in an osteochondroma of the pelvis. The chondrosarcoma has become so large as to obscure the original osteochondroma.

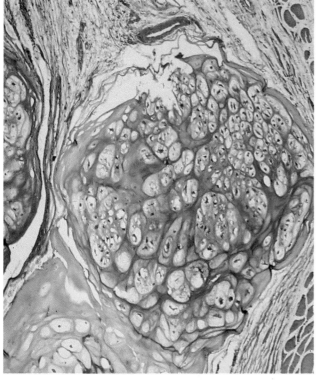

**Figure 16–10.** This low-power photomicrograph shows the invasion of skeletal muscle adjacent to the secondary chondrosarcoma.

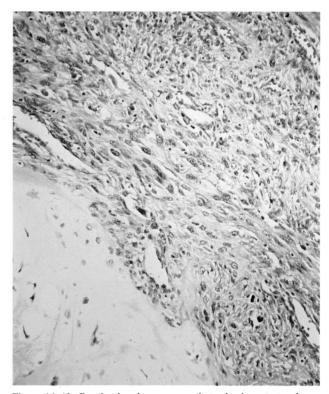

**Figure 16–12.** Rarely chondrosarcomas that arise in an osteochondroma may show foci of ''dedifferentiation,'' so-called secondary dedifferentiated chondrosarcoma. In this example of such a case, the characteristic pattern of hypercellular spindle cell tumor is superimposed on the low-grade hyaline cartilage malignancy that developed in an osteochondroma.

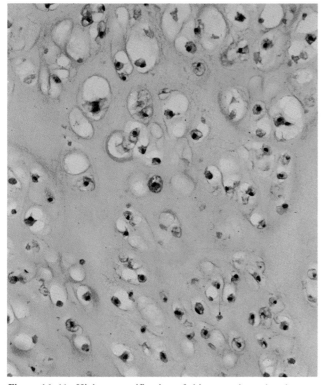

**Figure 16–11.** Higher magnification of this secondary chondrosarcoma shows the characteristic features of a low-grade hyaline cartilage malignancy: (1) hypercellularity, (2) pleomorphism, and (3) binucleation of the chondrocytes.

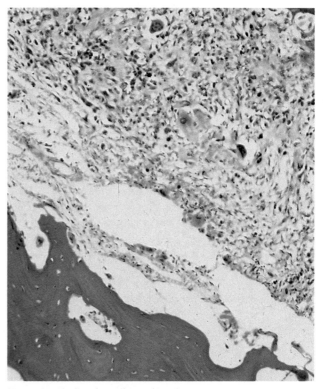

**Figure 16–13.** Rarely malignancies other than chondrosarcoma may arise in an osteochondroma. This photomicrograph shows an osteosarcoma that developed in an osteochondroma.

# CHAPTER 17

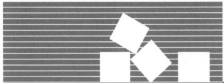

# Dedifferentiated Chondrosarcoma

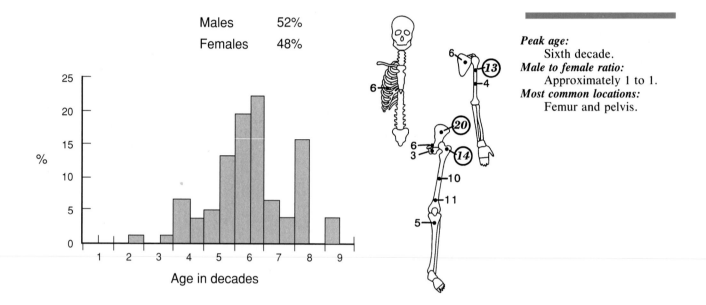

Males 52%
Females 48%

%

Age in decades

*Peak age:*
Sixth decade.
*Male to female ratio:*
Approximately 1 to 1.
*Most common locations:*
Femur and pelvis.

■ **Clinical Symptoms**

1. Pain is a universal symptom, and a mass lesion is frequently present.
2. Some long-standing indolent tumors may show an abrupt change in the pain pattern or accelerated growth of a mass lesion.

■ **Clinical Signs**

1. A soft tissue mass may be the only finding on physical examination.

■ **Major Radiographic Features**

1. An "aggressive" area is superimposed on what is otherwise typical of chondrosarcoma. This usually takes the form of radiolucent region but may also be a permeative destructive region within the tumor.
2. The lesion is often large and poorly marginated.

3. Intramedullary calcification of a cartilage tumor is usually present.
4. Cortical destruction and an associated soft tissue mass are evident.
5. Many cases are indistinguishable from ordinary intramedullary chondrosarcomas.

■ **Radiographic Differential Diagnosis**

1. Ordinary chondrosarcoma.
2. Sarcoma arising in an old infarct.
3. Mesenchymal chondrosarcoma.
4. Osteosarcoma.

■ **Pathologic Features**

*Gross*

1. This tumor shows a bimorphic gross appearance; areas of lobulated, gray-white hyaline cartilage coexist with regions of more fleshy, yellow-brown, soft tumor.

2. There is an abrupt transition from the hyaline cartilage component of the tumor, which is usually centrally located, to the spindle-cell component.
3. The anaplastic component of the tumor nearly always dominates the gross lesion and usually has caused cortical destruction of the affected bone with associated production of a soft tissue mass.

*Microscopic*

1. The grossly evident bimorphic pattern is also appreciable histologically.
2. The low-grade hyaline cartilage component shows the typical features of ordinary chondrosarcoma.
3. Immediately adjacent to the lobules of well-differentiated chondrosarcoma are sheet-like regions of high-grade spindle cell malignancy.
4. Osteoid matrix may be identified in the spindle cell component of the lesion.
5. The spindle cell component of the lesion may show the histologic features of fibrosarcoma or malignant fibrous histiocytoma.

## ■ Pathologic Differential Diagnosis

Benign lesions:
1. Chondroma, if incompletely sampled.
Malignant lesions:
1. Chondrosarcoma, ordinary type.
2. Osteosarcoma.
3. Fibrosarcoma.
4. Malignant fibrous histiocytoma.

## ■ Treatment

**Primary Modality:** Surgical ablation by amputation is usually necessary because of aggressive soft tissue invasion by the tumor.

**Other Possible Approaches:** limb-saving resection and oncologic reconstruction if an adequately wide margin can be achieved. Adjuvant chemotherapy protocols are currently being evaluated.

## References

Dahlin DC, and Beabout JW: Dedifferentiation of low-grade chondrosarcomas. Cancer 28:461–466, 1971.
McCarthy EF, and Dorfman HD: Chondrosarcoma of bone with dedifferentiation: a study of eighteen cases. Hum Pathol 13:36–40, 1982.
Mirra JM, and Marcove RC: Fibrosarcomatous dedifferentiation of primary and secondary chondrosarcoma: review of five cases. J Bone Joint Surg 56A:285–296, 1974.

**Figure 17–2.** The gross appearance of the lesion correlates well with the radiographic evidence of cortical destruction and associated soft tissue extension.

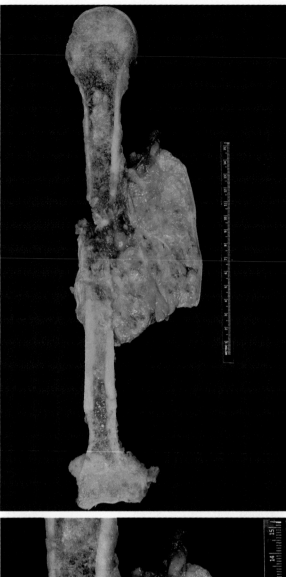

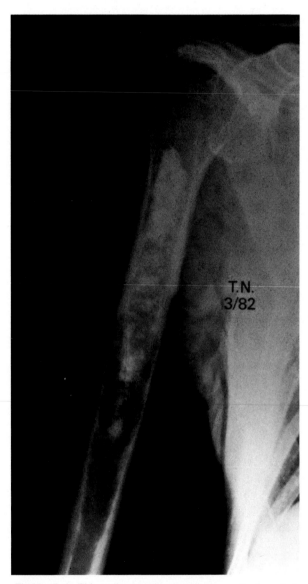

**Figure 17–1.** This radiograph illustrates a large diaphyseal dedifferentiated chondrosarcoma of the humerus. The aggressive destruction of the area, inferiorly superimposed on an otherwise typical appearance of chondrosarcoma, suggests the correct diagnosis.

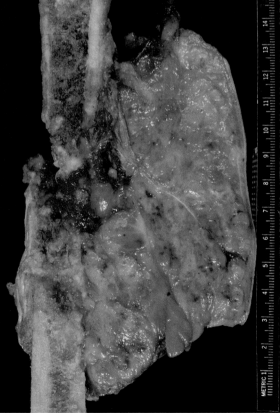

**Figure 17–3.** Although the majority of the lesion is fleshy and distinctly different grossly from the usual hyaline cartilage tumor, the medullary portion of the tumor shows the characteristic glistening blue-gray aura of the underlying low-grade chondrosarcoma.

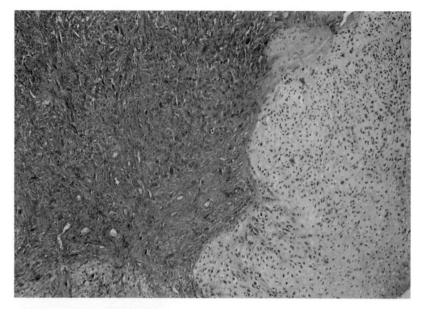

**Figure 17–4.** At low magnification, dedifferentiated chondrosarcoma shows a bimorphic pattern consisting of a hypocellular cartilage tumor juxtaposed with a high-grade spindle cell sarcoma.

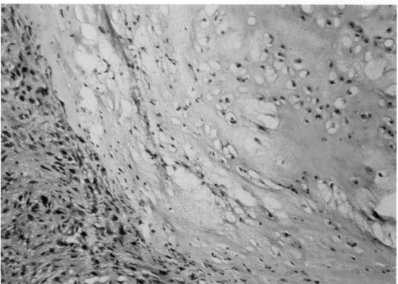

**Figure 17–5.** At higher magnification, the hyaline cartilage portion of the tumor is indistinguishable from a low-grade chondrosarcoma. In contrast, the hypercellular spindle cell portion of the tumor may be identical with a fibrosarcoma, malignant fibrous histiocytoma, or fibroblastic osteosarcoma.

**Figure 17–6.** At high magnification the cytologic atypia associated with the high-grade portion of the tumor is evident. Osteoid may be identified, as is shown in this photomicrograph.

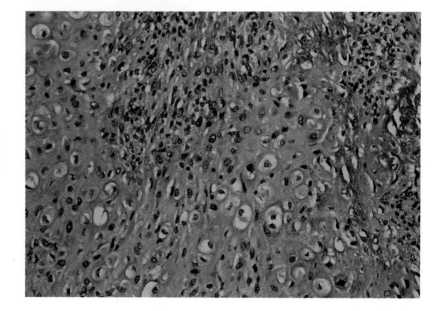

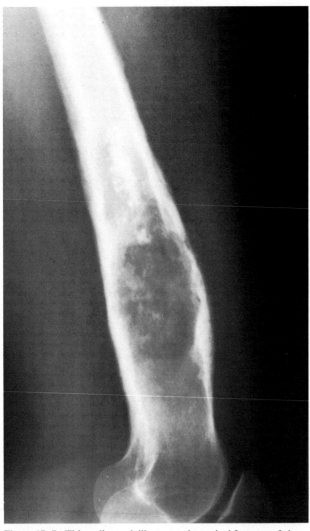

**Figure 17–7.** This radiograph illustrates the typical features of chondrosarcoma superiorly but shows a very aggressive appearance inferiorly, worrisome for a dedifferentiated chondrosarcoma.

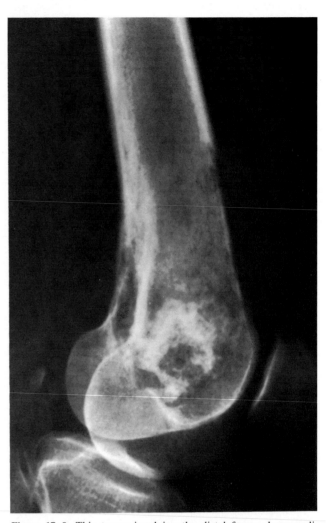

**Figure 17–9.** This tumor involving the distal femur shows radiographic features typical of chondrosarcoma distally. Again, however, a permeative destructive pattern of growth, seen proximally in the lesion, suggests that the tumor is a dedifferentiated chondrosarcoma.

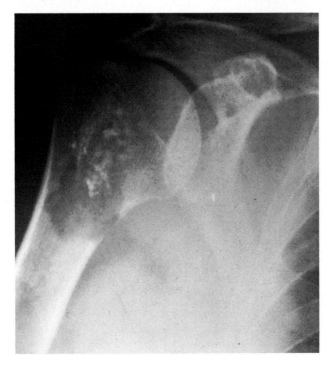

**Figure 17–8.** This dedifferentiated chondrosarcoma of the proximal humerus shows an aggressive lytic region inferiorly superimposed on an otherwise typical radiographic appearance for chondrosarcoma. The medial cortical destruction is particularly worrisome for dedifferentiation.

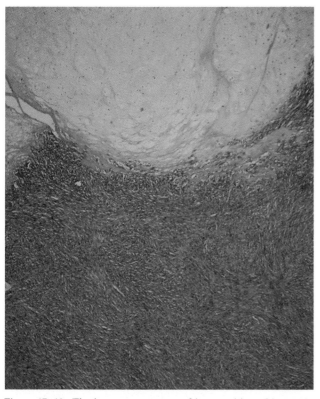

**Figure 17–10.** The low-power pattern of juxtaposition of hypocellular hyaline cartilage tumor and hypercellular spindle cell sarcoma is characteristic of dedifferentiated chondrosarcoma.

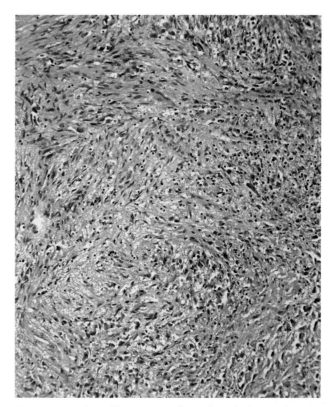

**Figure 17–12.** A storiform pattern of growth, as is characteristically associated with malignant fibrous histiocytoma, may also be seen in the dedifferentiated portion of the tumor.

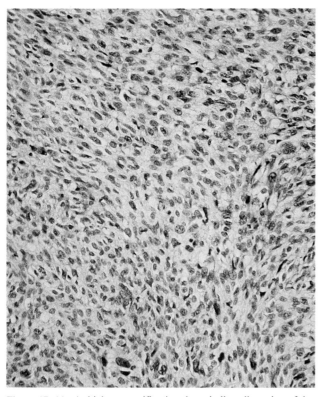

**Figure 17–11.** At higher magnification the spindle cell portion of the tumor may show a "herring-bone" pattern of growth, as is seen in fibrosarcoma.

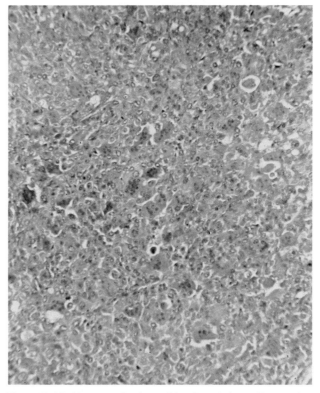

**Figure 17–13.** Numerous benign multinucleated giant cells may also be seen in the hypercellular portion of the tumor. Such a pattern may histologically mimic the appearance of malignant fibrous histiocytoma or malignant giant cell tumor.

# CHAPTER 18

## Mesenchymal Chondrosarcoma

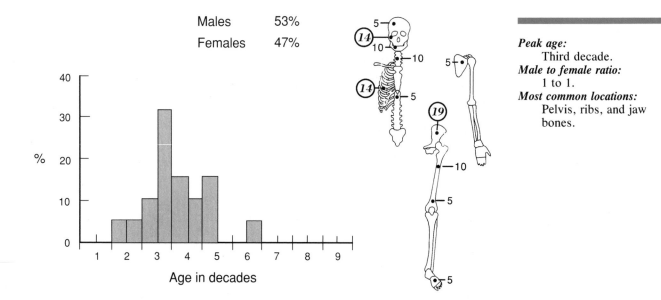

Males 53%
Females 47%

%

Age in decades

*Peak age:*
   Third decade.
*Male to female ratio:*
   1 to 1.
*Most common locations:*
   Pelvis, ribs, and jaw
   bones.

■ **Clinical Symptoms**

1. Pain and swelling are usually the only symptoms.
2. Approximately one-third of the patients have had symptoms of longer than one year's duration at the time of diagnosis.

■ **Clinical Signs**

1. A mass lesion is usually the only clinical sign.

■ **Major Radiographic Features**

1. Most mesenchymal chondrosarcomas have malignant radiographic appearance but no specific diagnostic features, or the radiographic features are suggestive of ordinary chondrosarcoma.
2. The tumor usually shows calcification.
3. Poor margination and cortical destruction are present.

4. Frequently there is an associated soft tissue mass.

■ **Radiographic Differential Diagnosis**

1. Chondrosarcoma.
2. Osteosarcoma.
3. Fibrosarcoma.

■ **Pathologic Features**

*Gross*

1. These tumors are typically gray to pink and vary from firm to soft in consistency.
2. The border of the tumor is usually well defined.
3. Hard calcific foci are usually scattered through the tumor.
4. Necrosis and hemorrhage may be evident.

*Microscopic*

1. The low-power pattern shows a bimorphic appearance with islands of benign-appearing hyaline cartilage embedded within highly cellular zones of small, round to slightly spindled cells.
2. Chondroid zones vary in size and may be more calcified or even ossified.
3. The pattern on low-power magnification in the cellular regions is usually hemangiopericytomatous in character, with numerous thin-walled branching vessels coursing through the tumor.
4. On higher magnification the cells within the cellular regions have uniform cytologic characteristics, being round to oval with uniform round to oval nuclei.

## ■ Pathologic Differential Diagnosis

Benign lesions:
1. Benign hemangiopericytoma.
Malignant lesions:
1. Ewing's sarcoma.
2. Dedifferentiated chondrosarcoma.
3. Osteosarcoma.
4. Malignant hemangiopericytoma.

## ■ Treatment

**Primary Modality:** surgical resection with a wide margin and reconstruction individualized to the location and the patient. This tumor's aggressive behavior with extensive involvement often mandates amputation to achieve an adequate margin.

**Other Possible Approaches:** Adjuvant chemotherapy protocols are being evaluated. Therapeutic radiation is indicated for surgically inaccessible lesions.

## References

Dabska M, and Huvos AG: Mesenchymal chondrosarcoma in the young: a clinicopathologic study of 19 patients with explanation of histogenesis. Virchows Arch (Pathol Anat) Histopathol *399*:89–104, 1983.

Huvos AG, Rosen G, Dabska M, and Marcove RC: Mesenchymal chondrosarcoma: a clinicopathologic analysis of 35 patients with emphasis on treatment. Cancer *51*:1230–1237, 1983.

Steiner GC, Mirra JM, and Bullough PG: Mesenchymal chondrosarcoma: a study of the ultrastructure. Cancer *32*:926–939, 1973.

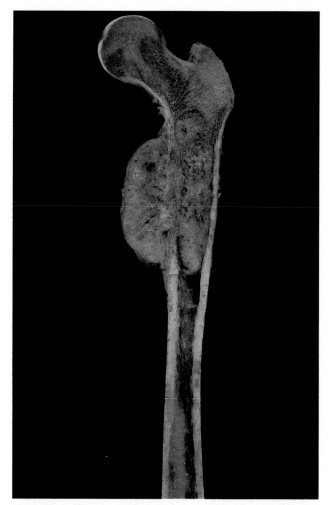

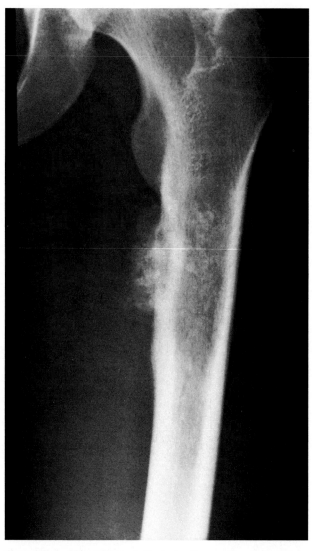

**Figure 18–2.** The gross pathologic features of the case correlate well with the radiographic appearance shown in Figure 18–1. The tumor is fleshy in quality, in contrast with a hyaline cartilage tumor. However, the lesional tissue may be gritty owing to foci of calcification within the tumor.

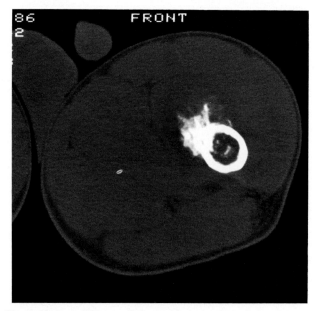

**Figure 18–1.** This radiograph illustrates the poorly marginated appearance of a mesenchymal chondrosarcoma. The lesion exhibits calcification, a feature suggesting that this is a cartilage tumor. The cortical destruction and associated soft tissue mass are radiographic indications of the malignancy of the process.

**Figure 18–3.** A CT scan of the tumor shows the soft tissue extent of the lesion as well as the medullary involvement.

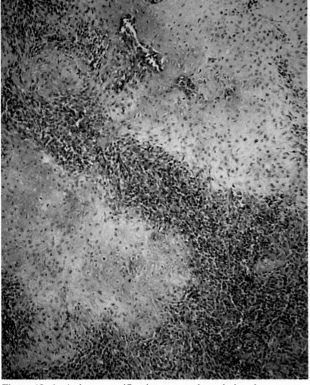

**Figure 18–4.** At low magnification mesenchymal chondrosarcomas are "bimorphic" tumors, composed of relatively hypocellular chondroid zones and hypercellular regions. The hypercellular regions consist of small cells.

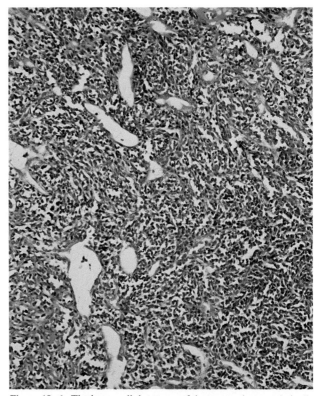

**Figure 18–6.** The hypercellular zones of the tumor characteristically have a hemangiopericytomatous pattern of growth, as is illustrated in this photomicrograph. "Stag horn"–like vascular spaces are evident at low magnification.

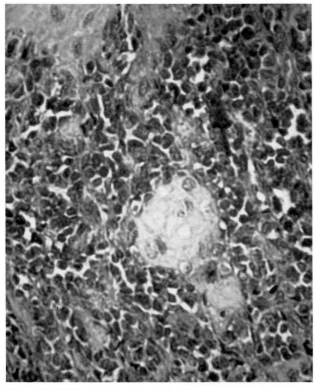

**Figure 18–5.** Chondroid zones within the tumor are variable in size, some being quite small as is shown in this photomicrograph.

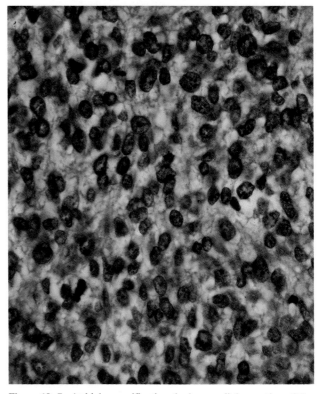

**Figure 18–7.** At high magnification the hypercellular portion of the tumor is composed of small cells, which are round to oval in shape. The cytologic features are similar to those of small-cell osteosarcoma and hemangiopericytoma.

**Figure 18–9.** This mesenchymal chondrosarcoma involves the acetabular region, a location often involved in ordinary chondrosarcoma. The bone shows lytic destruction, and there is associated calcification in the soft tissue portion of the tumor.

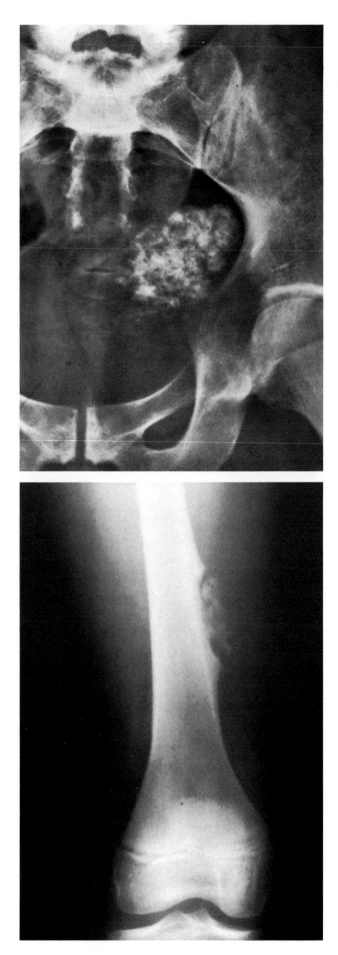

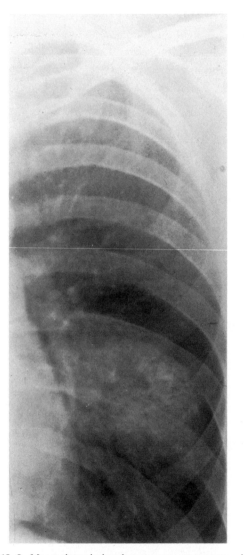

**Figure 18–8.** Mesenchymal chondrosarcomas are common in flat-bone locations, as in this case involving the rib. There is an associated large, partially calcified soft tissue mass with apparent underlying cortical destruction of the affected rib.

**Figure 18–10.** This periosteal tumor of the femoral diaphysis proved to be a mesenchymal chondrosarcoma. The buttresses and periosteal location are atypical of mesenchymal chondrosarcoma, as the majority of these lesions are centrally located.

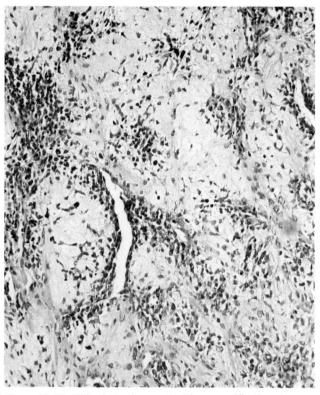

**Figure 18–11.** This photomicrograph at low magnification shows a mesenchymal chondrosarcoma in which the hyaline cartilage portion of the lesion predominates. The small-cell portion of the tumor persists in a perivascular pattern.

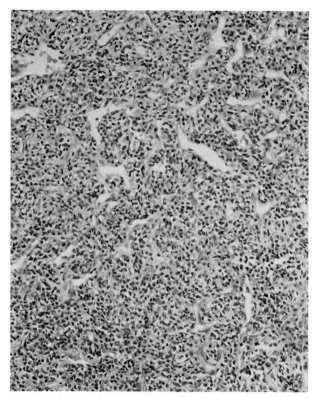

**Figure 18–13.** The hemangiopericytomatous pattern of growth is particularly prominent in this mesenchymal chondrosarcoma that involves the mandible, a common primary location for the tumor.

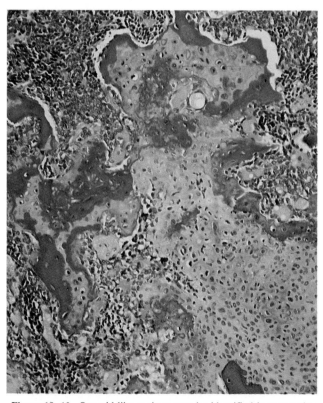

**Figure 18–12.** Osteoid-like regions may be identified in mesenchymal chondrosarcoma. The differential diagnosis in such cases includes small-cell osteosarcoma, a lesion that probably is closely related to mesenchymal chondrosarcoma.

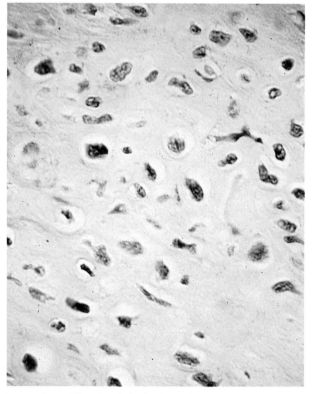

**Figure 18–14.** The chondroid portions of a mesenchymal chondrosarcoma are indistinguishable from ordinary chondrosarcoma. A small sample from such a region would be identified as an ordinary chondrosarcoma.

# CHAPTER 19

# Clear Cell Chondrosarcoma

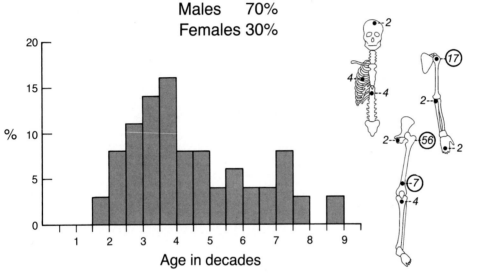

Males    70%
Females 30%

% — Age in decades

**Peak age:**
Third decade of life; however, the tumor is rare, and although none have occurred in the first decade, they have been seen in the ninth decade.

**Male to female ratio:**
2 to 1.

**Most common location:**
The proximal femur accounts for approximately 50 per cent of cases. The tumor nearly always involves the epiphyseal region of a long bone.

## ■ Clinical Symptoms

1. Pain is the most common symptom at the time of presentation.
2. These tumors are slow-growing; as such, the symptoms may be of long duration. Eighteen per cent of patients in the Mayo Clinic series had symptoms for longer than five years.

## ■ Clinical Signs

1. Regional tenderness is present.
2. A mass lesion may be found on physical examination.

## ■ Major Radiographic Features

1. The lesion has an epiphyseal location in the proximal femur or humerus.
2. Early lesions look benign with sharp margina-tion, sclerosis at the periphery, and expansion of the affected bone.
3. Twenty-five per cent are calcified on plain x-ray.
4. Larger lesions look malignant, with poor margination and cortical destruction.

## ■ Radiographic Differential Diagnosis

1. Chondroblastoma.
2. Chondrosarcoma, ordinary type.
3. Giant cell tumor.

## ■ Pathologic Features

### Gross

1. The curetted fragments are frequently found to contain a cartilaginous matrix of bluish-gray translucent matrix.
2. Cystic spaces may be identified; these may rep-

110

resent secondary aneurysmal bone cyst formation.

*Microscopic*

1. On low magnification these tumors are faintly
   lobulated and variable from region to region.
   Foci of obvious cartilage matrix production may
   lie adjacent to zones containing numerous mononuclear and multinucleated giant cells.
2. Bony trabeculae are usually identified in this
   tumor on low power. These are either at the center of lobules of tumor or scattered within the
   zones of mononuclear cells.
3. On higher magnification the tumor cells have ve-
   sicular nuclei and characteristically show abundant clear cytoplasm. The cell boundaries between such cells are usually distinct.
4. About 50 per cent of the tumors show regions of
   ordinary chondrosarcoma, and in these regions
   the multinucleated giant cells are not identified.

## ■ Pathologic Differential Diagnosis

Benign lesions:
1. Chondroblastoma.
2. Osteoblastoma.
3. Aneurysmal bone cyst.
Malignant lesions:
1. Chondrosarcoma, ordinary type.
2. Chondroblastic osteosarcoma.

## ■ Treatment

**Primary Modality:** en bloc resection with a wide
surgical margin and reconstruction of the joint by custom prosthesis, osteochondral allograft, or resection
arthrodesis, depending on the location and the needs
of the patient.

**Other Possible Approaches:** Amputation may be
necessary with large lesions, recurrent lesions, or lesions associated with local contamination due to a
pathologic fracture or where a wide margin cannot be
achieved with resection.

## References

Bjornsson J, Unni KK, Dahlin DC, et al: Clear cell chondrosarcoma
   of bone: observations in 47 cases. Am J Surg Pathol 8:223–230,
   1984.
Faraggiana T, Sender B, and Glicksman P: Light- and electron-microscopic study of clear cell chondrosarcoma. Am J Clin Pathol
   75:117–121, 1981.

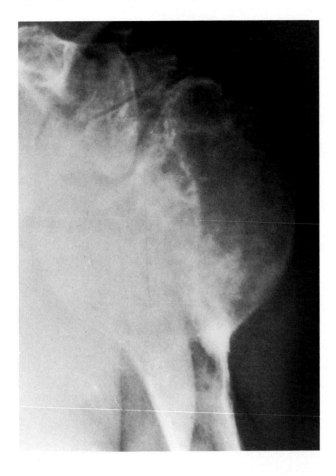

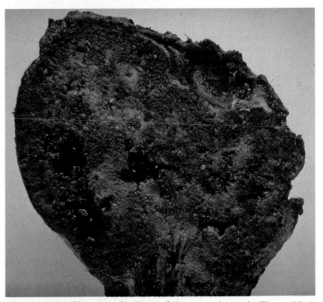

**Figure 19–1.** This radiograph shows a clear cell chondrosarcoma of the proximal humerus causing marked expansion of the bone and cortical thinning. Mottled calcification is present. At this point in the evolution of the tumor a radiographic diagnosis of chondrosarcoma, ordinary type, would be most likely. The radiographic features of the lesion 10 years earlier (see Fig. 19–3) are more characteristic of clear cell chondrosarcoma.

**Figure 19–2.** The gross features of the case shown in Figure 19–1 correlate well with its radiographic appearance. Hemorrhagic cystic spaces are evident in this tumor. Such regions of secondary aneurysmal bone cyst are frequently seen in cases of clear cell chondrosarcoma.

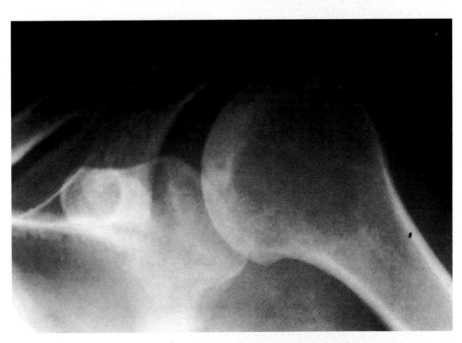

**Figure 19–3.** The margins of the clear cell chondrosarcoma are better defined in this radiograph of the proximal humerus 10 years prior to definitive surgery. There is only mild expansion of the bone, and no calcification is present. These radiographic features are nonspecific but suggestive of a benign lesion. Early in their evolution, clear cell chondrosarcomas frequently mimic benign conditions.

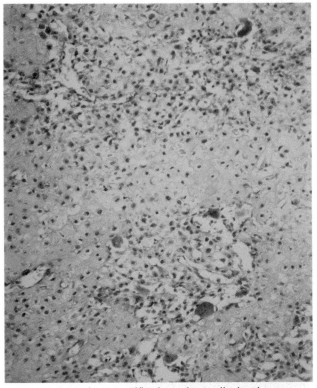

**Figure 19–4.** At low magnification, clear cell chondrosarcomas show a variable histologic pattern of growth. Hyaline cartilage regions interdigitate with more cellular regions, as is shown in this case involving the proximal femur.

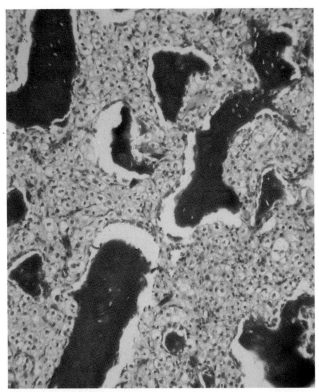

**Figure 19–6.** Clear cell chondrosarcoma will show an invasive pattern of growth at the periphery of the lesion. In this photomicrograph, permeation through the adjacent medullary bone is evident.

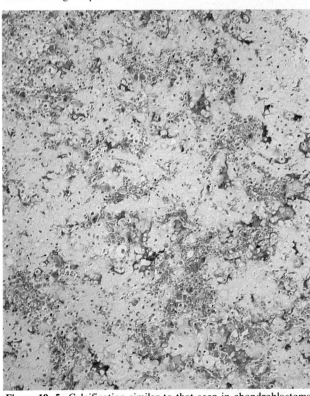

**Figure 19–5.** Calcification similar to that seen in chondroblastoma may be found in clear cell chondrosarcoma. This feature, in combination with the histologic variability and the presence of benign multinucleated giant cells, may result in a mistaken diagnosis of chondroblastoma.

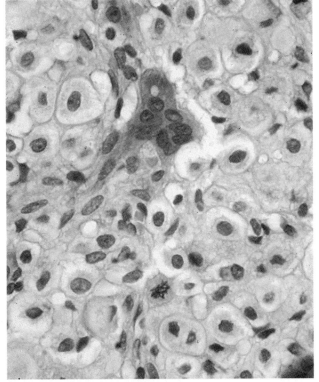

**Figure 19–7.** At high magnification the cytologic features of clear cell chondrosarcoma may be deceptively bland. Tumor cells show abundant cytoplasm, as is illustrated in this photomicrograph. The presence of such polygonal cytoplasm, bland nuclear features, and the presence of multinucleated giant cells mimic the features of chondroblastoma.

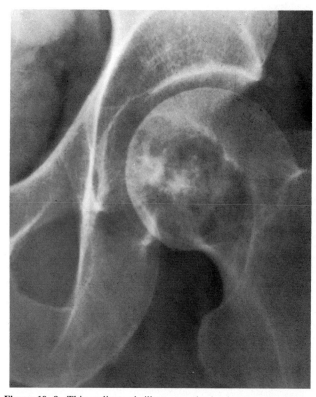

**Figure 19–8.** This radiograph illustrates the benign features commonly seen in cases of clear cell chondrosarcoma. The sharp sclerotic margin of this tumor is compatible with the appearance of chondroblastoma.

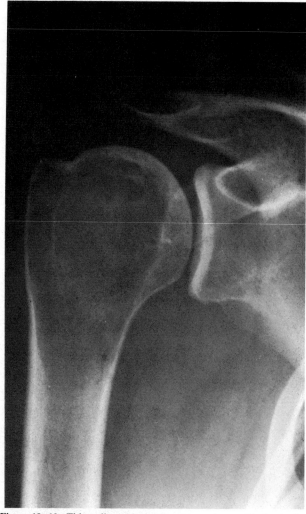

**Figure 19–10.** This radiograph shows a more advanced lesion in the proximal humerus, presenting as a purely lytic and poorly marginated tumor.

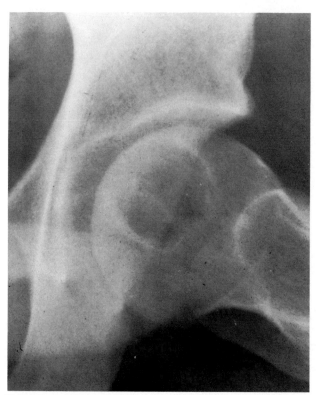

**Figure 19–9.** Like chondroblastoma, clear cell chondrosarcoma frequently involves the epiphysis of the affected bone. Such is the case in this tumor, which is partially calcified, has sclerotic margins, and involves the epiphysis of the proximal femur.

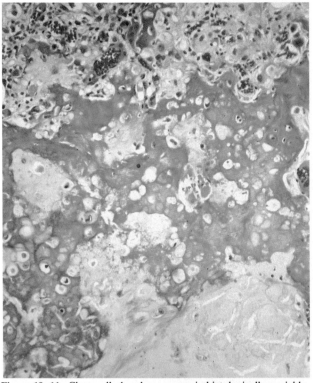

**Figure 19–11.** Clear-cell chondrosarcoma is histologically variable from region to region, as is shown in this low-power photomicrograph. Foci may show pure hyaline cartilage differentiation whereas other regions may show bone production. Thus the differential diagnosis may include ordinary chondrosarcoma as well as chondroblastic osteosarcoma.

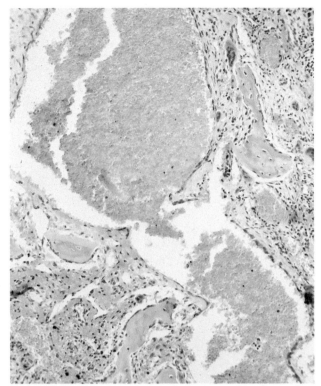

**Figure 19–13.** This photomicrograph shows a region of secondary aneurysmal bone cyst complicating clear cell chondrosarcoma. Although such secondary aneurysmal bone cysts are more commonly encountered in benign tumors, they are quite frequently seen as a component in clear cell chondrosarcoma.

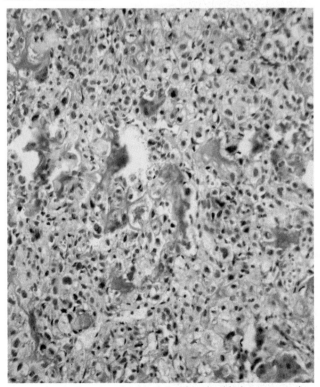

**Figure 19–12.** Bone production is evident in this low-power photomicrograph. Such foci may mimic the appearance of a chondroblastic osteosarcoma. However, the cytologic atypia is much less pronounced in clear cell chondrosarcoma than in chondroblastic osteosarcoma.

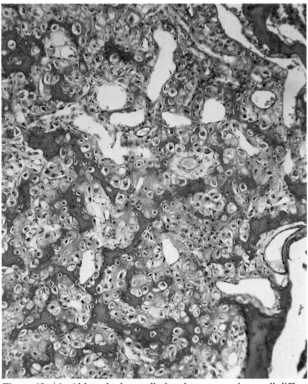

**Figure 19–14.** Although clear cell chondrosarcoma is a well-differentiated or low-grade tumor, it can recur locally or in other osseous locations or metastasize to the lung. The histologic features of the pulmonary metastases are identical with the primary tumor, as is illustrated in this photomicrograph.

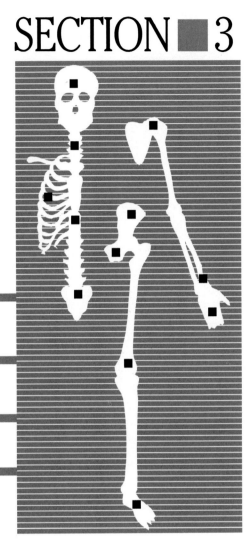

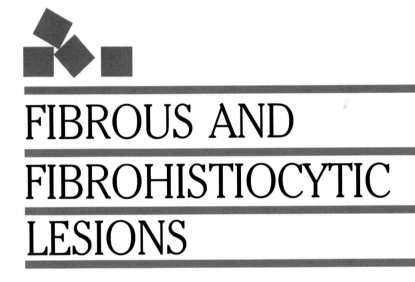

# FIBROUS AND FIBROHISTIOCYTIC LESIONS

# CHAPTER 20

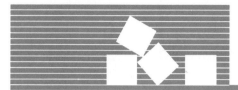

# Fibrous Dysplasia

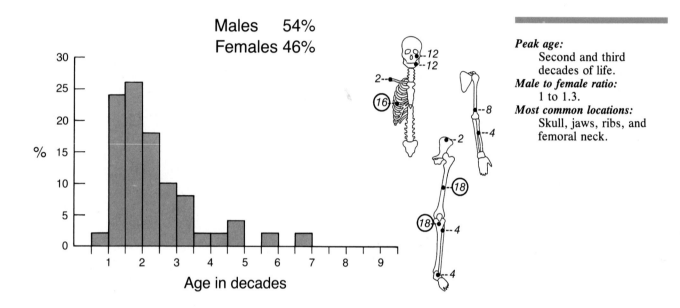

Males    54%
Females 46%

%

30
25
20
15
10
5
0

1  2  3  4  5  6  7  8  9

Age in decades

**Peak age:**
  Second and third
  decades of life.
**Male to female ratio:**
  1 to 1.3.
**Most common locations:**
  Skull, jaws, ribs, and
  femoral neck.

## ■ Clinical Symptoms

1. Most patients are asymptomatic.
2. Abnormal bone growth may result in deformity.
3. Pain may be present.
4. Swelling may be noted; when the process involves the skull bones, the patient may present with exophthalmos.
5. Involvement of the femoral neck may result in weakening and resultant pathologic fracture.

## ■ Clinical Signs

1. A localized swelling may be found.
2. Exophthalmos may be present if skull bones are involved.
3. Cutaneous pigmentation may be seen, associated with polyostotic disease (Albright's syndrome).
4. Precocious puberty in girls may be associated with polyostotic disease (Albright's syndrome).

5. Soft tissue myxomas have been reported in association with fibrous dysplasia ("Mazabraud's" syndrome).

## ■ Major Radiographic Features

1. The lesion is metaphyseal or diaphyseal in location.
2. It is usually lytic or ground glass–like in density.
3. The affected bone shows expansion and sharp margination of the lesion.
4. Bowing and pathologic fracture may be seen.
5. The lesion may be surrounded by a thick rind of sclerotic bone.
6. Multiple bones may be affected (polyostotic).

## ■ Radiographic Differential Diagnosis

1. Fibroma (metaphyseal fibrous defect, nonossifying fibroma).

2. Unicameral bone cyst (simple cyst).
3. Chondromyxoid fibroma.
4. Aneurysmal bone cyst.

## ■ Pathologic Features

### Gross

1. Lesional tissue is usually dense and fibrous.
2. Osteoid trabeculae within the fibrous tissue imparts a gritty quality to the lesion when it is cut.
3. Prominent cyst formation may be present; such cysts are most commonly filled with a clear, yellowish fluid.
4. Dense ossification may also occur within the lesional tissue.

### Microscopic

1. At low magnification the lesion is composed of proliferating fibroblasts that produce a dense collagenous matrix.
2. Osteoid trabeculae course irregularly through the connective tissue.
3. The trabeculae are arranged in a haphazard, nonfunctional manner, and they may contain reversal lines mimicking the appearance of Paget's disease.
4. A metaplastic chondroid component may be present and rarely is so prominent as to raise the question of whether the lesion represents a hyaline cartilage neoplasm.
5. Cystic degeneration may be identified. These regions of degeneration may also show numerous lipophages and benign multinucleated giant cells. Rarely the lesion shows marked myxoid change.
6. At higher magnification no cytologic atypia is seen.

## ■ Pathologic Differential Diagnosis

Benign lesions:
1. Paget's disease.
2. Giant cell reparative granuloma.
Malignant lesions:
1. Low-grade central osteosarcoma.
2. Parosteal osteosarcoma (if the location is not known).

## ■ Treatment

**Primary Modality:**   observation if the lesion is asymptomatic.

**Other Possible Approaches:**   curettage and grafting or resection.

### References

Campanacci M, and Laus M: Osteofibrous dysplasia of the tibia and fibula. J Bone Joint Surg 63A:367–375, 1981.

Nager, GT, Kennedy DW, and Kopstein E: Fibrous dysplasia: a review of the disease and its manifestations in the temporal bone. Ann Otol Rhinol Laryngol (Suppl) 92:1–52, 1982.

Nakashima Y, Yamamuro T, Fumiwara Y, et al: Osteofibrous dysplasia (ossifying fibroma of long bones): a study of 12 cases. Cancer 52:909–914, 1983.

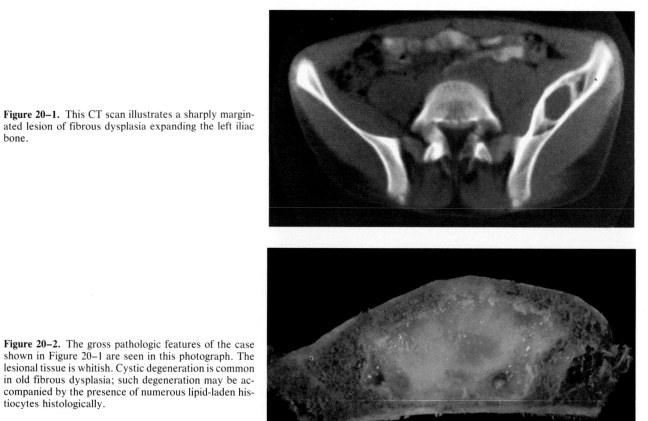

**Figure 20–1.** This CT scan illustrates a sharply margin-ated lesion of fibrous dysplasia expanding the left iliac bone.

**Figure 20–2.** The gross pathologic features of the case shown in Figure 20–1 are seen in this photograph. The lesional tissue is whitish. Cystic degeneration is common in old fibrous dysplasia; such degeneration may be ac-companied by the presence of numerous lipid-laden his-tiocytes histologically.

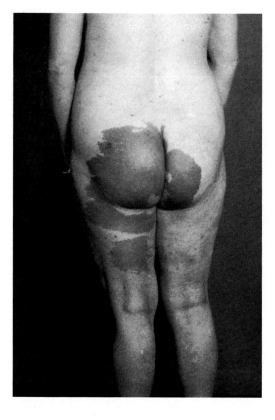

**Figure 20–3.** Pigmentation, as shown in this photograph, may be seen in cases of Albright's syndrome (polyostotic fibrous dysplasia).

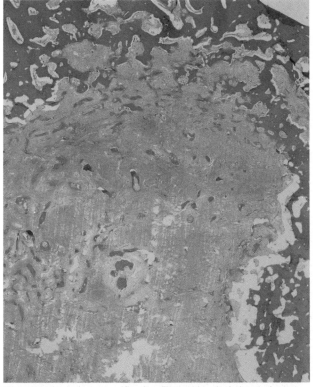

**Figure 20–4.** At low magnification fibrous dysplasia is relatively hypocellular and composed of a spindle cell stroma, within which numerous irregular trabeculae of osteoid are present.

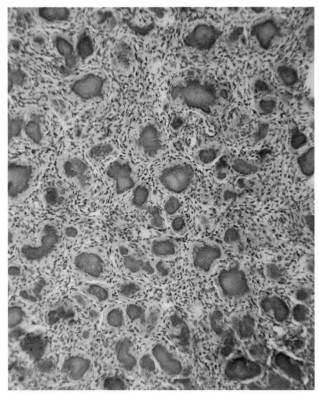

**Figure 20–6.** Occasionally the osteoid produced in fibrous dysplasia may mimic the appearance of cementum or even psammomatous calcification, as is seen in a meningioma. Such is the case in this lesion of the ilium.

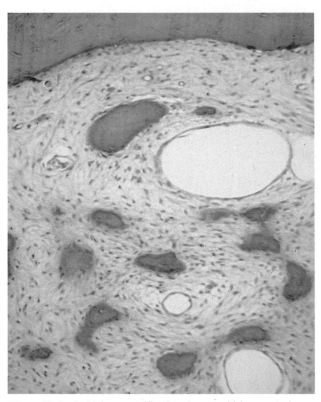

**Figure 20–5.** At higher magnification the osteoid is seen to be arranged in a nonfunctional manner. The shape of the osteoid may be irregular or round to oval, as is seen in this case of fibrous dysplasia involving the rib.

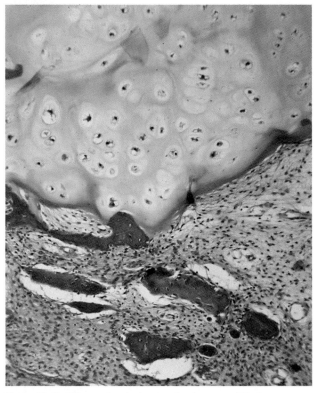

**Figure 20–7.** Fibrous dysplasia may also have a cartilaginous component; in such cases the designation of fibrocartilaginous dysplasia is appropriate. This example of such a lesion was taken from the femur of a patient with Albright's syndrome.

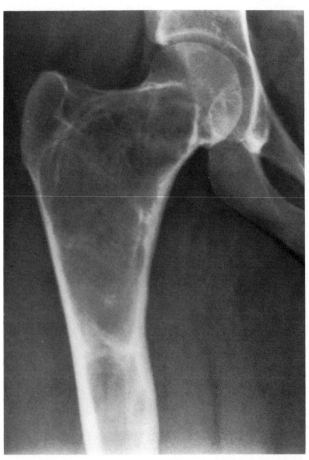

**Figure 20–8.** The proximal femur is a common location for fibrous dysplasia. This lesion, which has resulted in extensive expansion of the proximal femur, shows the sharp margination and sclerotic rim associated with a benign process.

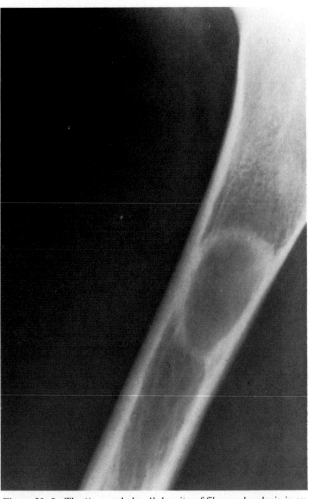

**Figure 20–9.** The "ground glass" density of fibrous dysplasia is evident in this radiograph of a lesion involving the medulla of the femur. Note the thick rind of surrounding sclerosis.

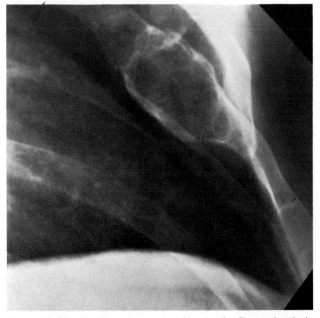

**Figure 20–10.** The ribs are a common location for fibrous dysplasia. This example shows expansion of the affected rib, commonly seen in such cases, and sclerosis of the surrounding bone.

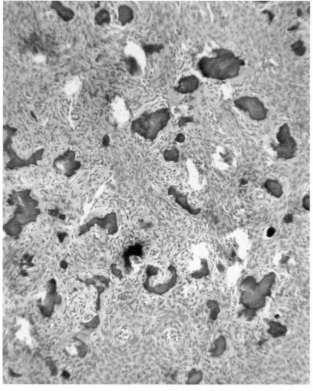

**Figure 20–11.** Fibrous dysplasia may involve the flat bones of the skull, as in this case. In such cases, the irregular psammoma body–like ossification of the lesion may result in a pattern simulating that of a meningioma secondarily involving the affected bone.

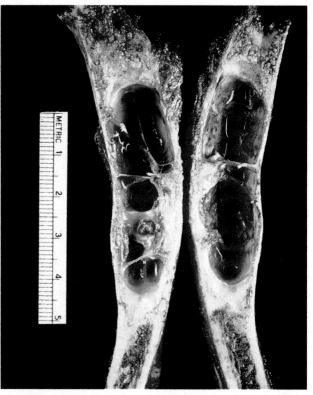

**Figure 20–13.** Cystic degeneration is a feature most commonly associated with fibrous dysplasia of the rib, as is seen in this case.

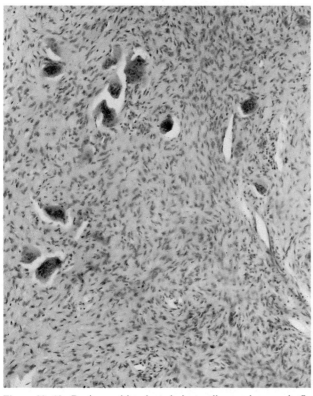

**Figure 20–12.** Benign multinucleated giant cells may be seen in fibrous dysplasia, as in this case involving the humerus. Like other lesions that contain numerous giant cells, the lesion may be confused with giant cell tumor and other giant cell–containing bone lesions.

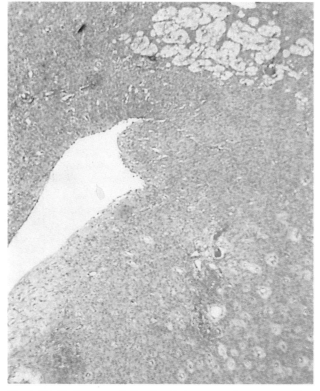

**Figure 20–14.** ''Foam cells'' or lipid-laden macrophages are another indication of a degenerative process. Such foci are evident in this example of fibrous dysplasia involving the proximal femur.

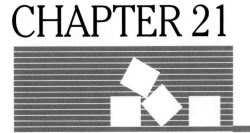

# CHAPTER 21

# Benign and Atypical Fibrous Histiocytoma

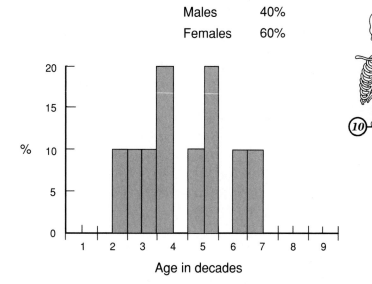

Males 40%
Females 60%

%

Age in decades

**Peak age:**
Generally reported in adulthood, but this lesion is extremely uncommon.

**Male to female ratio:**
1 to 1.5.

**Most common location:**
Occurs in nonmetaphyseal locations and has most frequently been reported in flat bones, e.g., the ilium.

■ **Clinical Symptoms**

1. Local pain is the most common symptom associated with these lesions.
2. A mass may be found if the lesion involves a superficial bone.

■ **Clinical Signs**

1. These lesions are generally asymptomatic, and there are no findings that are common on physical examination.

■ **Major Radiographic Features**

1. The lesion is lytic, without matrix mineralization.
2. It has a sharp margin, often with a sclerotic rim and expansion of the affected bone.

3. Larger lesions may destroy the cortex and extend into soft tissues, suggesting a malignant process.

■ **Radiographic Differential Diagnosis**

1. Fibroma.
2. Fibrous dysplasia.
3. Chondromyxoid fibroma.

■ **Pathologic Features**

*Gross*

1. Curetted fragments have most frequently been described as firm.
2. Lesional tissue varies in color from red-brown to yellow, as does the tissue of a fibroma.

*Microscopic*

1. The light-microscopic appearance of this lesion is identical with that of a fibroma.
2. At low magnification a storiform arrangement of the spindling cells is evident.
3. Hemosiderin and lipid-laden histiocytes are commonly identifiable.
4. At higher magnification the tumor shows a uniform cytologic appearance of the nuclei, and mitotic figures are rare.

## ■ Pathologic Differential Diagnosis

Benign lesions:
1. Fibroma (metaphyseal fibrous defect).
2. Giant cell tumor of tendon sheath type.
3. Pigmented villonodular synovitis.

Malignant lesions:
1. Malignant fibrous histiocytoma.

## ■ Treatment

**Primary Modality:**   curettage and bone grafting.
**Other Possible Approaches:**   Lesions with a favorable location, such as the ilium, may be removed by en bloc resection with a marginal or wide margin when this can be performed without significant loss of function.

## References

Bertoni F, Capanna R, Calderoni P, and Bacchini P: Case report 223. Skeletal Radiol 9:215–217, 1983.

Fechner RE: Benign fibrous histiocytoma of bone (abstract). Lab Invest 52:21A, 1985.

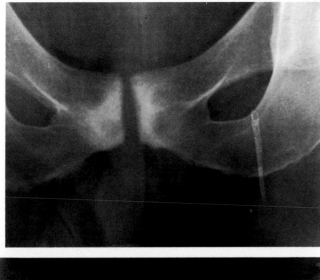

A

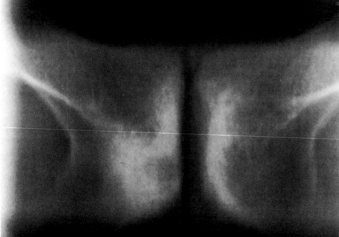

B

**Figure 21–1.** This radiograph (*A*) and tomogram (*B*) illustrate a benign fibrous histiocytoma of the pubis. A small, oval lytic tumor with sharp margination and surrounding sclerosis indicates the benign nature of the process.

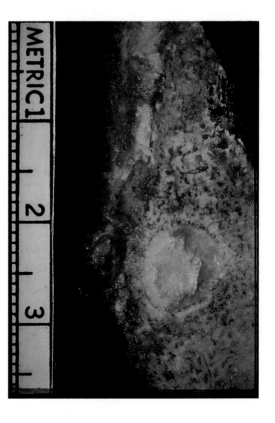

**Figure 21–2.** This gross photograph illustrates the well-circumscribed, fibrous appearance of a benign fibrous histiocytoma involving the pubis.

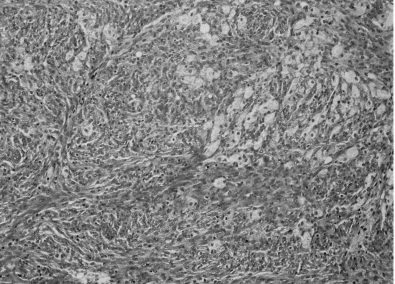

**Figure 21–3.** Histologically, benign fibrous histiocytomas are indistinguishable from metaphyseal fibrous defects (fibromas). This lesion from the tibia of a 28-year-old female shows the admixture of lipid-laden histiocytes and spindle cells, which may be arranged in a storiform pattern.

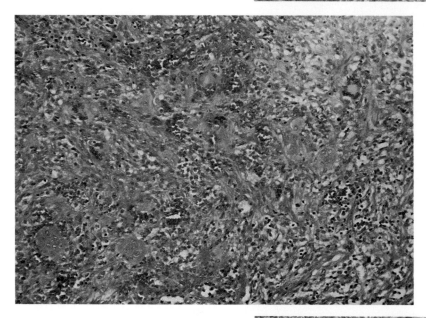

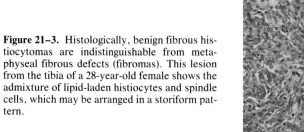

**Figure 21–4.** Multinucleated giant cells, as illustrated in this photomicrograph, are commonly seen in cases classified as benign fibrous histiocytoma. This tumor was in the sacrum.

**Figure 21–5.** Like fibromas, benign fibrous histiocytomas show variability from region to region. This region in a lesion from the sacrum contains few lipid-laden cells and no giant cells.

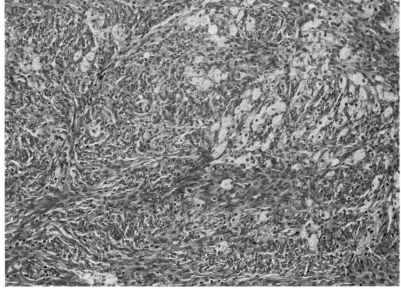

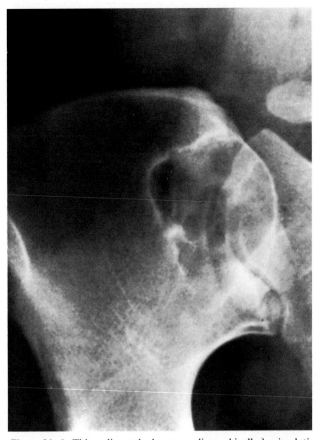

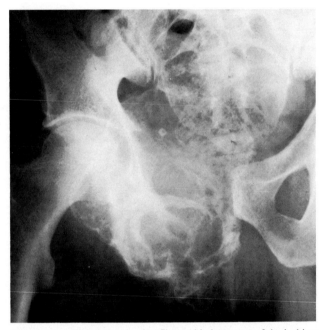

**Figure 21–6.** This radiograph shows a radiographically benign lytic lesion of the iliac bone. The sharp margination, expansion, and sclerotic rim support a benign diagnosis. The lesion was found to represent a benign fibrous histiocytoma on biopsy.

**Figure 21–7.** This large, benign fibrous histiocytoma of the ischium and pubis shows cortical destruction and soft tissue extension.

# CHAPTER 22

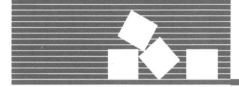

# Fibrosarcoma

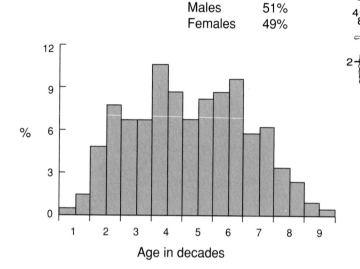

Males 51%
Females 49%

%

Age in decades

*Peak age:*
Broad age range with minor peaks in the fourth and sixth decades.
*Male to female ratio:*
1 to 1.
*Most common locations:*
Distal femur and proximal tibia, with the femur accounting for approximately 25 per cent of all cases.

## ■ Clinical Symptoms

1. Pain and swelling are common, as with all malignant bone tumors.
2. The duration of symptoms is generally short.
3. Fibrosarcoma may arise "secondarily" in a precursor lesion such as a bone infarct or in Paget's disease, but the most common precursor condition is radiation therapy.

## ■ Clinical Signs

1. A mass lesion is generally present in the area of the affected bone.
2. The mass is generally painful to palpation.

## ■ Major Radiographic Features

1. The lesion is large and eccentrically located.
2. The lesion may be metaphyseal or diaphyseal within the affected bone.

3. The lesion is purely lytic with sclerosis absent or scant.
4. The lesion is poorly marginated.
5. Cortical destruction and extension into the adjacent soft tissues are common.
6. A periosteal reaction is uncommonly seen.
7. Approximately 30 per cent arise secondarily in a preexisting lesion.

## ■ Radiographic Differential Diagnosis

1. Osteosarcoma.
2. Myeloma.
3. Metastatic carcinoma.
4. Giant cell tumor.
5. Malignant fibrous histiocytoma.

## ■ Pathologic Features

*Gross*

1. The lesional tissue is firm and fleshy.

2. Myxoid qualities may be present, and high-grade tumors may be grossly hemorrhagic, friable, and necrotic.
3. Most tumors will have broken through the cortex.

*Microscopic*

1. At low magnification the histologic view is classically that of a spindle cell tumor arranged in a "herring bone" pattern of growth.
2. At its periphery, the lesion grows in a permeative manner, invading between preexisting bony trabeculae.
3. Low-grade tumors may produce abundant collagen and may be relatively hypocellular.
4. High-grade tumors are more cellular, showing less collagen production.
5. On high magnification the cytologic features vary with the grade of the tumor. Low-grade tumors show homogeneous cytologic features with dark, spindle-shaped nuclei; high-grade tumors show marked nuclear pleomorphism and abundant mitotic activity.
6. Rarely the tumor may be markedly myxoid.

## ■ Pathologic Differential Diagnosis

Benign lesions:
1. Desmoplastic fibroma.

Malignant lesions:
1. Malignant fibrous histiocytoma.
2. Fibroblastic osteosarcoma.
3. Metastatic spindling carcinoma.

## ■ Treatment

**Primary Modality:** preoperative chemotherapy and limb-sparing resection with a wide surgical margin and reconstruction as indicated, where feasible. However, amputation may be required to achieve an adequate margin. The adjuvant multidrug chemotherapy programs, similar to those used for osteosarcoma, are currently being evaluated.

**Other Possible Approaches:** radiation therapy for surgically inaccessible lesions and aggressive thoracotomy for pulmonary metastases.

## References

Larsson SE, Lorentzon R, and Boquist L: Fibrosarcoma of bone: a demographic, clinical and histopathological study of all cases recorded in the Swedish Cancer Registry From 1958 to 1968. J Bone Joint Surg *58B*:412–417, 1976.

Sugiura I: Desmoplastic fibroma: case report and review of the literature. J Bone Joint Surg *58A*:126–130, 1976.

Taconis WK, and Van Rijssel TG: Fibrosarcoma of long bones: a study of the significance of areas of malignant fibrous histiocytoma. J Bone Joint Surg *67B*:111–116, 1985.

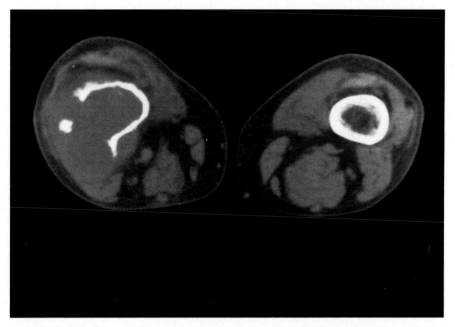

**Figure 22–1.** This CT scan shows a large lytic and eccentric defect in the distal femur. Cortical destruction and soft tissue extension of the lesion attest to its malignant nature; however, the tumor is otherwise nondescript.

**Figure 22–2.** The gross pathologic features of the fibrosarcoma in Figure 22–1 are shown in this photograph. The lesional tissue is soft and gray-white to tan in color. The cortical destruction and soft tissue extension evident radiographically are illustrated grossly in this cross-section of the tumor.

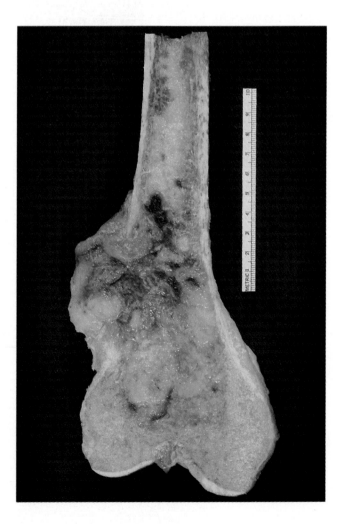

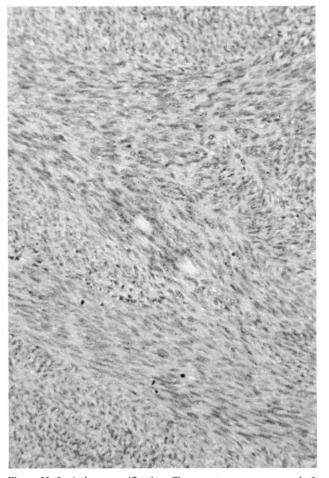

**Figure 22–3.** At low magnification, fibrosarcomas are composed of spindle cells arranged in a "herring-bone" pattern of growth. The high-grade tumors show greater cellularity, mitotic activity, and cytologic pleomorphism.

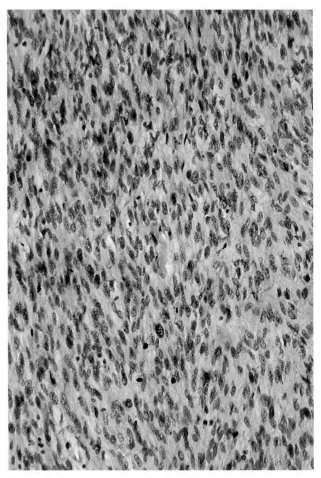

**Figure 22–4.** At higher magnification, fibrosarcomas vary in their degree of cytologic atypia and mitotic activity. This tumor that involved the maxilla resulted in pulmonary metastasis 34 months after diagnosis, attesting to its high-grade nature.

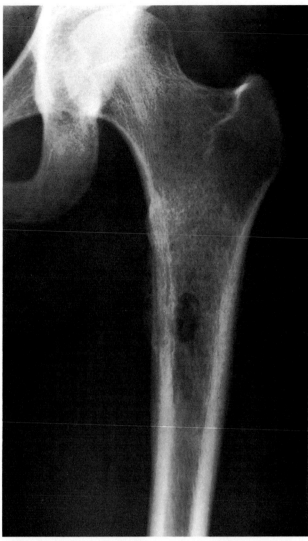

Figure 22–5. This radiograph shows a poorly marginated lytic fibrosarcoma in the subtrochanteric diaphyseal region of the femur. Scanty periosteal reaction is present in this case.

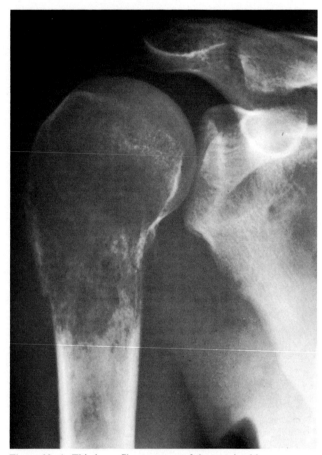

Figure 22–6. This large fibrosarcoma of the proximal humerus presented as a purely lytic metaphyseal lesion. The cortical destruction present attests to the aggressiveness of the lesion, and the bone has been sufficiently weakened to have sustained a pathologic fracture.

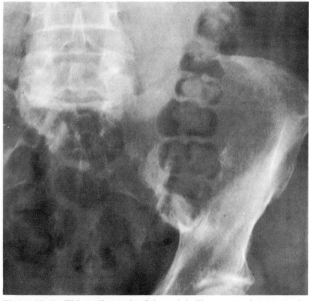

Figure 22–7. This radiograph of the pelvis illustrates a large, purely lytic fibrosarcoma of the left iliac bone and sacrum. There is extensive destruction of the bone.

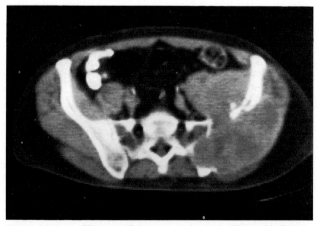

Figure 22–8. A CT scan of the tumor shown in Figure 22–7 demonstrates a large soft tissue component containing low-density areas of necrotic tumor or hemorrhage.

134

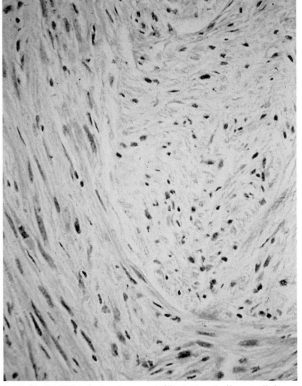

**Figure 22–9.** This photomicrograph illustrates the hypocellular nature of well-differentiated or low-grade fibrosarcomas. Although nuclear pleomorphism may be present, such tumors lack significant mitotic activity and generally show abundant collagenous stroma.

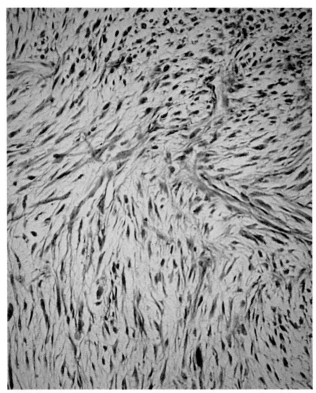

**Figure 22–11.** Myxoid stromal change may be present and generally accompanies low-grade fibrosarcomas.

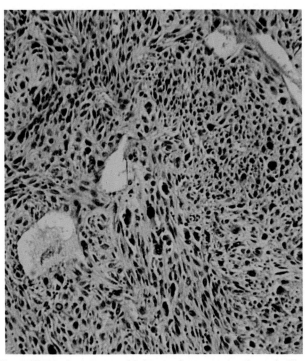

**Figure 22–10.** In contrast with low-grade tumors (as shown in Fig. 22–9), high-grade tumors are hypercellular and show less collagenous matrix production. Greater nuclear pleomorphism is also evident even at low magnification, as in this example of a high-grade fibrosarcoma.

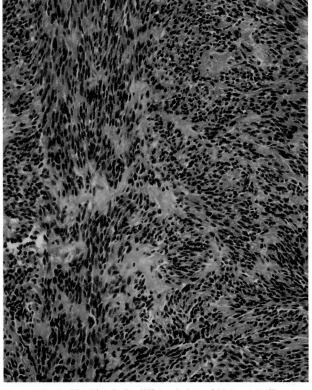

**Figure 22–12.** The histologic differentiation of high-grade fibrosarcoma from fibroblastic osteosarcoma is made on the basis of osteoid being identified in the osteosarcoma. However, dense collagen can mimic the appearance of osteoid, as is shown in this photomicrograph; thus the separation is at times subjective.

# CHAPTER 23

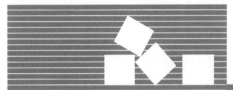

# Malignant Fibrous Histiocytoma

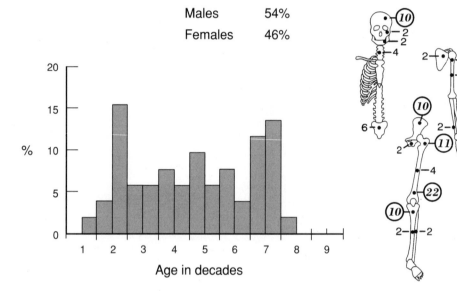

Males 54%
Females 46%

%

Age in decades

**Peak age:**
    Broad age range but
    more common in adults.
**Male to female ratio:**
    1 to 1.
**Most common location:**
    Distal femur.

■ **Clinical Symptoms**

1. Pain and swelling are the most common symptoms.
2. Symptoms may be of short duration but are generally present for six months or longer.
3. This tumor may arise after radiation therapy for an unrelated malignancy or as a malignancy complicating Paget's disease.

■ **Clinical Signs**

1. A painful or tender mass lesion is the most common finding on physical examination.

■ **Major Radiographic Features**

1. The lesion most often arises in a metaphyseal or diaphyseal location in the affected bone.
2. The lesion most often is purely lytic, although a few have mixed sclerosis and lysis.

3. Cortical destruction and associated soft tissue mass are common.
4. Periosteal reaction is absent or scant.
5. The tumor may be identified arising from a pre-existing lesion, e.g., a bone infarct.

■ **Radiographic Differential Diagnosis**

1. Osteosarcoma.
2. Fibrosarcoma.
3. Malignant lymphoma.
4. Metastatic carcinoma.
5. Myeloma.

■ **Pathologic Features**

*Gross*

1. The gross tumor varies in consistency from firm to soft, depending upon the cellularity and the amount of collagen being produced.

2. The color varies from tumor to tumor and within a given tumor; it may be yellow, brown, or tan.
3. Necrotic regions are frequently present in high-grade tumors.

### Microscopic

1. At low magnification the appearance is generally that of a spindle cell tumor arranged in a matted or storiform pattern.
2. The cytologic features tend to be quite variable, with some cells being more rounded and "histiocytic" and others spindled and "fibroblastic."
3. Multinucleated giant cells, lipid-laden histiocytes, and malignant giant cells are scattered throughout the lesion.
4. At higher magnification the cytologic atypia can be quite variable from low-grade to high-grade tumors, as can the variability in the mitotic activity present.

### ■ Pathologic Differential Diagnosis

Benign lesions:
1. Fibroma (metaphyseal fibrous defect).
2. Benign fibrous histiocytoma.
3. Giant cell tumor of tendon sheath or pigmented villonodular synovitis.
4. Giant cell tumor.
5. Giant cell reparative granuloma (giant cell reaction).

Malignant lesions:
1. Metastatic sarcomatoid carcinoma (particularly hypernephroma).
2. Fibrosarcoma.
3. Fibroblastic osteosarcoma.

### ■ Treatment

**Primary Modality:**  preoperative chemotherapy and wide surgical resection when possible. Oncologic reconstruction varies with the location. Amputation may be necessary to achieve a margin in large lesions with neurovascular involvement.

**Other Possible Approaches:**  Adjuvant chemotherapy protocols are being evaluated. Thoracotomy is useful for patients with pulmonary metastases. Radiation therapy has been effective in some surgically inaccessible lesions.

### References

Capanna R, Bertoni F, Bacchini P, et al: Malignant fibrous histiocytoma of bone: The experience at the Rizzoli Institute: report of 90 cases. Cancer 54:177–187, 1984.

Ghandur-Mnaymneh L, Zych G, and Mnaymneh W: Primary malignant fibrous histiocytoma of bone: report of six cases with ultrastructural study and analysis of the literature. Cancer 49:698–707, 1982.

McCarthy EF, Matsuno T, and Dorfman HD: Malignant fibrous histiocytoma of bone: a study of 35 cases. Hum Pathol 10:57–70, 1979.

Mirra JM, Gold RH, and Marafiote R: Malignant (fibrous) histiocytoma arising in association with a bone infarct in sickle-cell disease: coincidence or cause and effect? Cancer 39:186–194, 1977.

Taconis WK, and Mulder JD: Fibrosarcoma and malignant fibrous histiocytoma of long bones: radiographic features and grading. Skeletal Radiol 11:237–245, 1984.

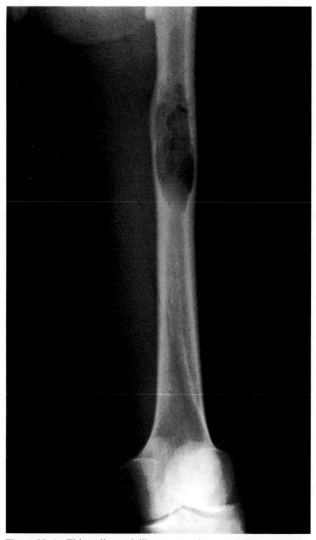

**Figure 23–1.** This radiograph illustrates an intramedullary malignant fibrous histiocytoma that shows a purely lytic pattern of growth. Mild expansion of the femoral diaphysis and cortical destruction are evident.

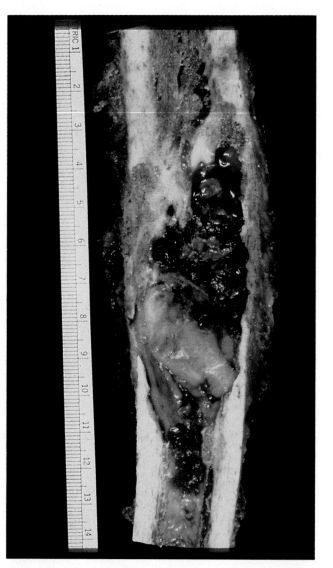

**Figure 23–2.** The gross pathologic features of this lesion correlate well with its radiographic appearance in Figure 23–1. The tumor is grossly soft, fleshy, and variable in color from gray-white to yellow. Foci of hemorrhage, as are visible in this case, may be present.

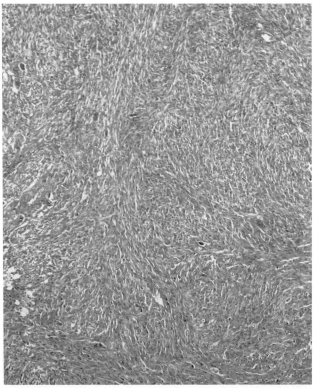

**Figure 23–3.** At low magnification, the histologic pattern of malignant fibrous histiocytoma may vary from region to region. Classically the tumor grows in a storiform pattern, as is shown in this photomicrograph.

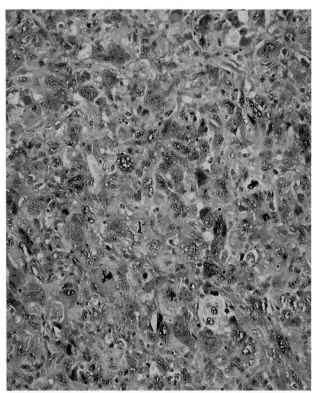

**Figure 23–5.** At higher magnification, the degree of cytologic atypia present in malignant fibrous histiocytomas is variable. Most commonly, significant cytologic atypia and brisk mitotic activity are present, as is shown in this photomicrograph.

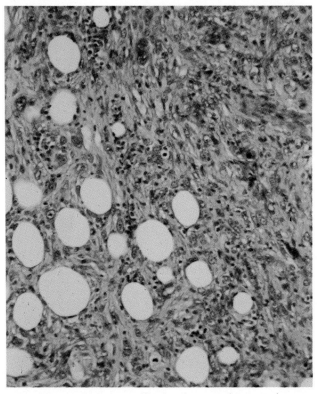

**Figure 23–4.** At higher magnification the tumor is seen to be composed of a variety of cell types. Some tumors have a pronounced inflammatory component; others show lesser degrees of inflammatory reaction.

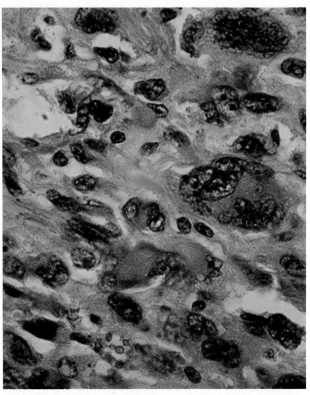

**Figure 23–6.** At high magnification, marked cytologic atypia characterized by nuclear pleomorphism, hyperchromasia, and an irregular chromatin pattern are common in malignant fibrous histiocytoma. Multinucleation is also common. Such tumors may simulate a giant cell tumor.

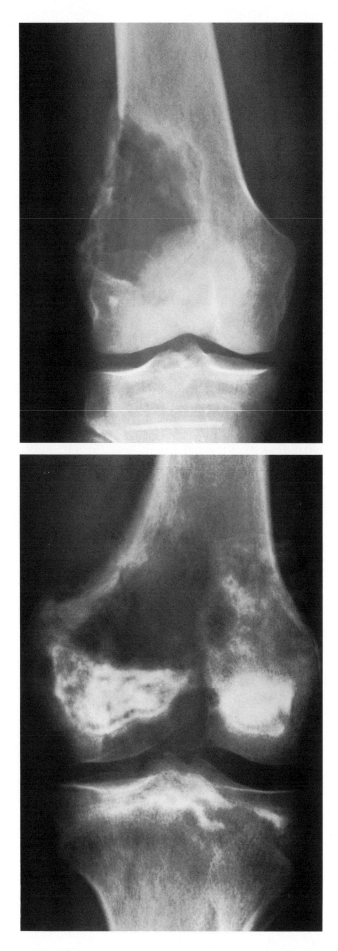

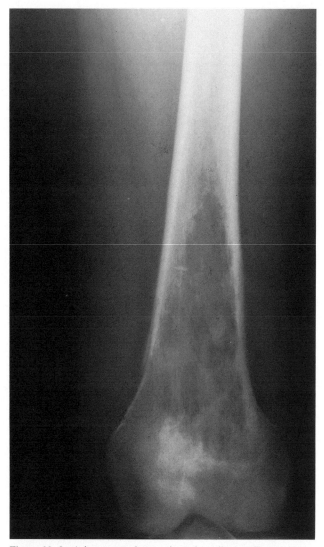

**Figure 23–7.** This radiograph illustrates a malignant fibrous histiocytoma of the distal femoral metaphysis. The tumor is eccentric and shows a permeative pattern of growth with cortical destruction.

**Figure 23–8.** A large, poorly marginated, malignant fibrous histiocytoma of the lower femoral diametaphysis is shown in this radiograph. The lesion is irregular in contour and shows a mixed lytic and sclerotic pattern of growth.

**Figure 23–9.** Malignant fibrous histiocytoma may arise secondary to a bone infarct, as is shown in this radiograph of the distal femur. Infarct is also present in the upper tibia.

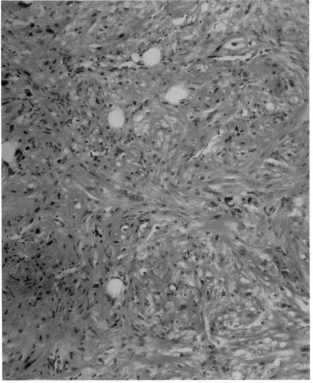

**Figure 23–10.** At low magnification, an ill-defined storiform pattern of growth is evident in this malignant fibrous histiocytoma of the proximal tibia. The tumor is growing in a permeative manner.

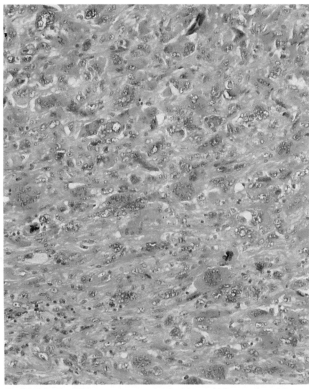

**Figure 23–12.** When numerous multinucleated giant cells are found in a tumor, careful assessment of the cytologic features of the mononuclear cells is necessary. At high magnification, the mononuclear cells of malignant fibrous histiocytoma are cytologically different from those of the multinucleated giant cells, as this photomicrograph shows.

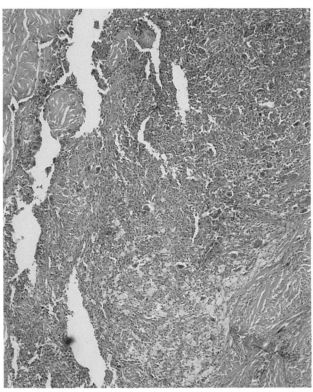

**Figure 23–11.** Numerous multinucleated giant cells may be present in malignant fibrous histiocytomas, resulting in a histologic appearance simulating that of giant cell tumor. This photomicrograph illustrates such a histologic pattern in a tumor that involved the distal femur.

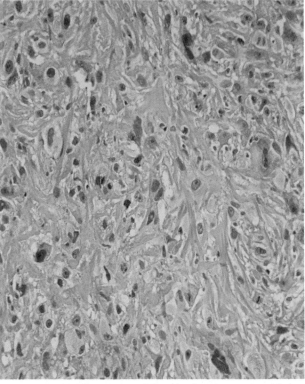

**Figure 23–13.** Differentiation of fibroblastic osteosarcoma (shown in this photomicrograph) from malignant fibrous histiocytoma can be extremely difficult. Demonstration of "malignant" osteoid in the lesion identifies it as an osteosarcoma; however, fracture callus and reactive new bone formation associated with malignant fibrous histiocytoma may simulate such osteoid. Such a distinction is probably only of academic importance.

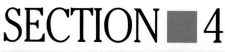

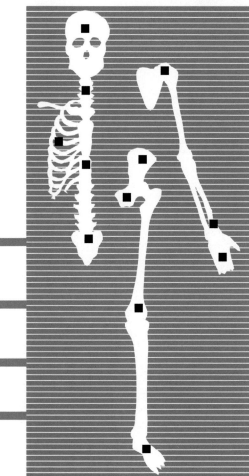

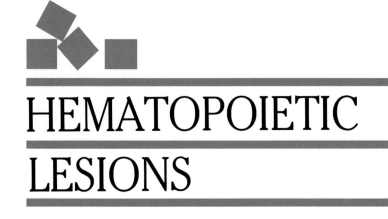

# HEMATOPOIETIC
# LESIONS

# CHAPTER 24

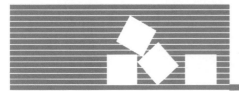

# Malignant Lymphoma

Males     62%
Females   38%

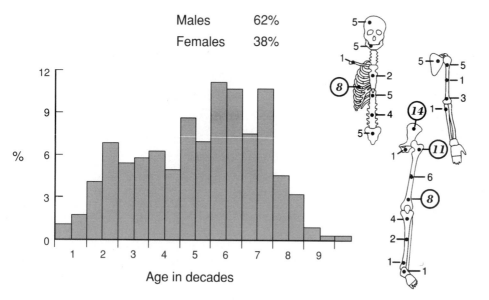

% / Age in decades

**Peak age:**
Broad age range with peak in the sixth and seventh decades of life.
**Male to female ratio:**
1.5 to 1.
**Most common location:**
May involve any bone or multiple bones, but the femur is involved in 25 per cent of cases.

■ **Clinical Symptoms**

1. Malignant lymphoma most commonly is associated with pain and swelling.
2. Pain is variable in intensity but may have been present for years.
3. Neurologic symptoms may be present in those patients who have vertebral involvement related to cord or nerve root compression.
4. The patient may have few complaints, however, and generally feels quite well despite extensive disease.

■ **Clinical Signs**

1. A tender mass lesion is commonly found on physical examination if the affected bone is superficial.
2. Lymphadenopathy and splenomegaly may be present in disseminated disease.

3. Extension into the soft tissues may result in an associated soft tissue mass.

■ **Major Radiographic Features**

1. The lesion is generally characterized by extensive diaphyseal permeative destruction of the affected bone.
2. The pattern may be one of pure lysis or sclerosis, or it may be a mixture of lysis and sclerosis.
3. Periosteal reaction is unusual.
4. The cortex may be thickened, and the lesion shows poor margination at the periphery.
5. An associated soft tissue mass is commonly present.
6. Isotope bone scan, computed tomography (CT), and magnetic resonance imaging (MRI) are frequently helpful in defining the extent of the lesion and its location.

144

## ■ Radiographic Differential Diagnosis

1. Ewing's sarcoma.
2. Osteosarcoma.
3. Osteomyelitis.
4. Metastatic carcinoma.

## ■ Pathologic Features

### Gross

1. Viable tumor extending into the soft tissues generally shows a whitish, fish flesh–like appearance.
2. Lymphomas generally permeate the bone extensively, leaving residual bony trabeculae that may impart a gritty consistency to the medullary portion of the specimen.

### Microscopic

1. At low magnification lymphomas show a diffuse sheet-like proliferation of cells without matrix production.
2. At higher magnification osseous lymphomas generally show a mixture of cells, with both small and large cells scattered throughout the lesional tissue.
3. The nuclear characteristics are generally quite variable, with both cleaved and noncleaved nuclei identifiable.
4. Reticulin stains will generally show a fine meshwork of reticulin fibers surrounding individual cells.
5. Immunohistochemical stains for lymphoid markers are positive if optimally fixed tissue is available for analysis. (Note: Touch preparations may be used for immunohistochemical analysis, thereby avoiding the use of tissue that has been subjected to decalcification procedures.)

## ■ Pathologic Differential Diagnosis

Benign lesions:
1. Chronic osteomyelitis.
Malignant lesions:
1. Metastatic undifferentiated carcinoma.
2. Malignant fibrous histiocytoma (histiocytic variant).

## ■ Treatment

**Primary Modality:** Radiation therapy is the mainstay of treatment of the local bony lesion. Chemotherapy is used when systemic disease is identifiable.

**Other Possible Approaches:** surgical intervention with internal fixation or joint replacement for pathologic fractures. Resection or amputation may be required for distal extremity lesions that have failed to respond to radiation therapy.

### References

Dosoretz DE, Murphy GF, Raymond AK, et al: Radiation therapy for primary lymphoma of bone. Cancer *51*:44–46, 1983.

Dosoretz DE, Raymond AK, Murphy GF, et al: Primary lymphoma of bone: the relationship of morphologic diversity to clinical behavior. Cancer *50*:1009–1014, 1982.

Reimer RR, Chabner BA, Young RC, et al: Lymphoma presenting in bone: results of histopathology, staging and therapy. Ann Intern Med *87*:50–55, 1977.

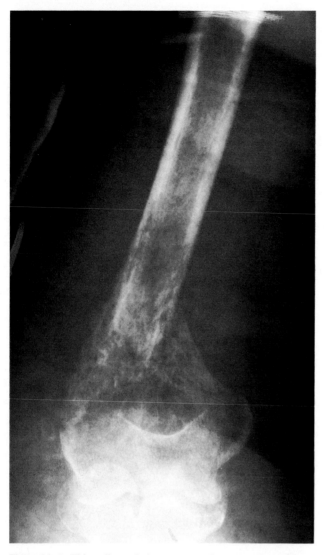

**Figure 24–1.** This radiograph demonstrates the permeative destructive appearance of a malignant lymphoma involving the distal humerus. An associated soft tissue mass is present, and a pathologic fracture has occurred.

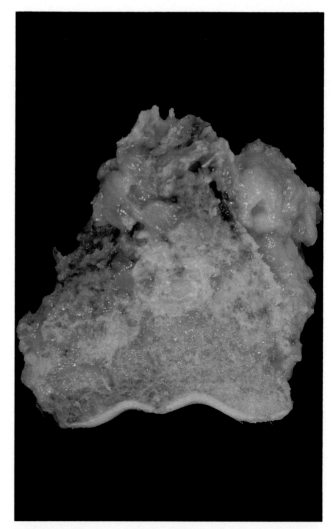

**Figure 24–2.** The gross pathologic features of malignant lymphoma of bone are demonstrated in this tumor, which was resected owing to the pathologic fracture and loss of bone. Classically lymphomas are soft, "fish flesh" tumors that are gray-white in color.

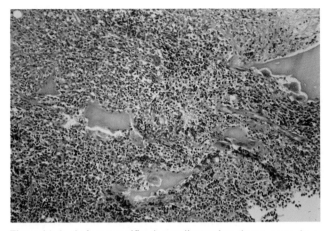

**Figure 24–3.** At low magnification malignant lymphoma grows in a permeative pattern, whether it involves bone (as in this photomicrograph) or soft tissue. Residual bony trabeculae are present within the medullary portion of this non-Hodgkin's lymphoma.

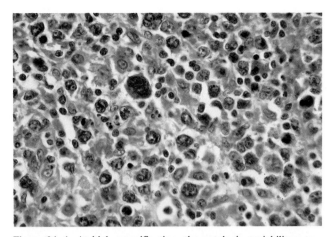

**Figure 24–4.** At high magnification, the cytologic variability generally present in osseous lymphomas is seen in this photomicrograph. Large and small cells are mixed and generally grow in a sheet-like, diffuse manner. "Multilobulated" cells may be seen, as in this example, and some cases represent neoplasms of T-cell origin; however, most osseous lymphomas are of B-cell lineage.

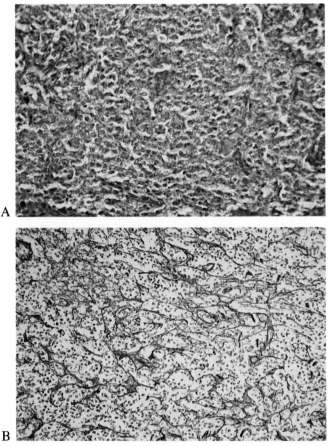

**Figure 24–5.** Special stains may be helpful in separating malignant lymphoma from other "small round cell" tumors. The periodic acid–Schiff stain (A) helps to distinguish lymphoma from Ewing's sarcoma, as lymphomas are negative and most Ewing's sarcomas are positive. Lymphomas may show more reticulin fibers (B, reticulin stain) than do Ewing's sarcomas.

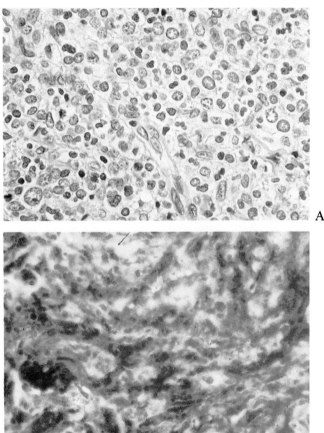

**Figure 24–6.** Other hematopoietic neoplasms may mimic the appearance of lymphoma. Granulocytic sarcoma is particularly notorious for resembling a diffuse mixed cell lymphoma, as is shown in A. Special stain may be helpful in separating such cases from lymphoma. The chloroacetate esterase stain (B) is positive in granulocytic sarcomas and negative in lymphomas.

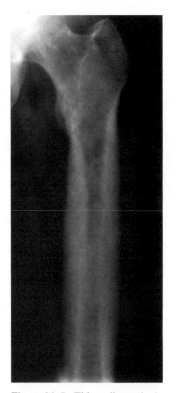

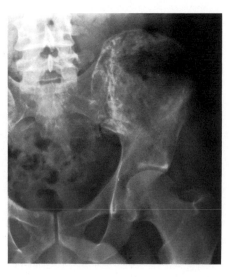

**Figure 24–8.** Although many lymphomas of bone show a lytic pattern radiographically, mixed lytic and sclerotic lesions, as shown in this tumor of the ilium, are common. The irregular, permeative pattern of growth of the tumor also favors a malignant process radiographically.

**Figure 24–7.** This radiograph shows an extensive diaphyseal lymphoma of the femur with poor margination and cortical thickening.

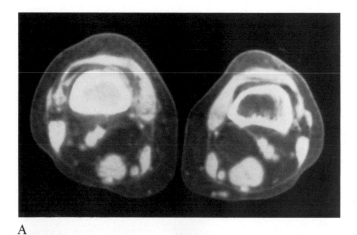

A

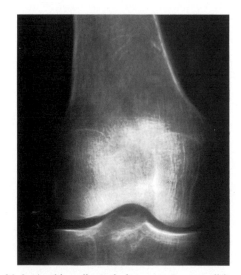

**Figure 24–9.** As this radiograph demonstrates, not all lymphomas are identifiable with plain x-ray. This patient had a tumor involving the distal femur.

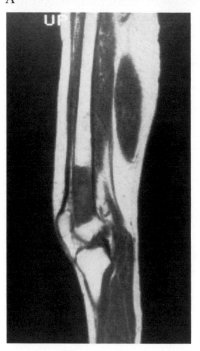

B

**Figure 24–10.** *A*, A CT scan of the distal femur seen in Figure 24–9 shows an intramedullary lymphoma. The radiographic density of the marrow in the right femur is greater than in the uninvolved left femur. MRI may also be helpful in such cases; in *B* the longitudinal extent of the lymphoma appears as a low-signal (black) area as compared with the normal marrow (white) in this sagittal reconstruction.

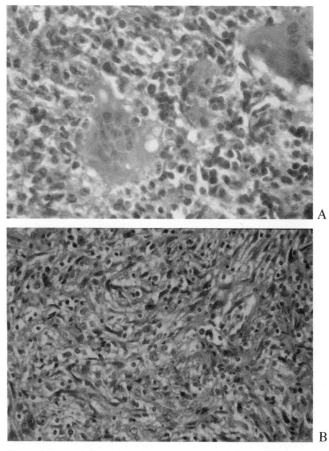

A

B

**Figure 24–13.** Malignant lymphoma can mimic other primary sarcomas of bone. *A* shows the presence of multinucleated giant cells in a lymphoma. The "histiocytic" appearance of the large cells in lymphoma and the presence of multinucleated giant cells may suggest the diagnosis of malignant fibrous histiocytoma. Although spindling of the cells is rare in lymphoma, such change may rarely be seen in osseous lymphomas (*B*) and may mimic histologically the appearance of a primary sarcoma.

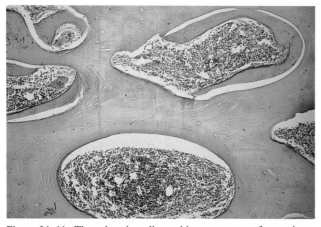

**Figure 24–11.** The sclerotic radiographic appearance of some lymphomas is due to the sclerotic reaction induced by the tumor. Such bony sclerosis is illustrated in this low-power photomicrograph of a calvarial lymphoma showing a permeative pattern of growth.

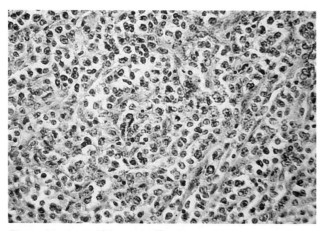

**Figure 24–12.** At higher magnification lymphomas generally are seen to be composed of a pleomorphic discohesive infiltrate, as is the case with this femoral tumor.

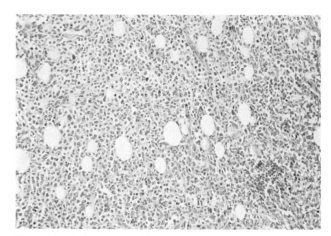

**Figure 24–14.** At low magnification, malignant lymphoma tends to grow in a permeative pattern that leaves behind parts of the normal architecture. The normal elements left may be bony trabeculae or fatty marrow elements, as this photomicrograph shows.

# CHAPTER 25

# Myeloma

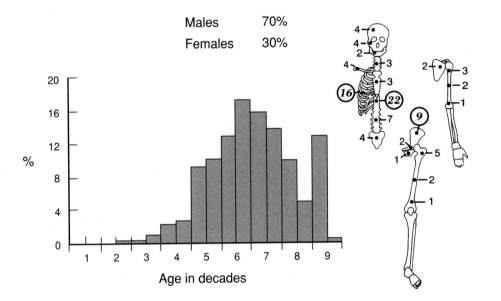

Males 70%
Females 30%

**Peak age:**
Sixth decade of life, and rare in patients less than 40 years of age.
**Male to female ratio:**
Approximately 2 to 1.
**Most common locations:**
Vertebra, ribs, and pelvis at the time of initial diagnosis, but the skull is usually involved at the time of death.

## ■ Clinical Symptoms

1. Pain is the most frequent complaint at the time of diagnosis.
2. The duration of the pain is usually less than six months.
3. Constitutional symptoms of weakness and weight loss are almost uniformly present.
4. Pathologic fracture results in a sudden onset of pain in many patients.
5. Peripheral neuropathy may be present, particularly in osteosclerotic myeloma.
6. A tendency toward bleeding and fever may also be experienced.

## ■ Clinical Signs

1. Local pain and tenderness are common on physical examination.
2. A palpable mass may be found due to extraos-

seous extension of the tumor or hemorrhage related to it.
3. Peripheral neuropathy may be detected in some patients.
4. Hypercalcemia occurs in less than 50 per cent of patients.
5. Hypergammaglobulinemia may manifest itself as rouleaux formation appreciable on peripheral blood smear.
6. Serum electrophoresis and immunoelectrophoresis generally reveal a monoclonal gammopathy, but nonsecretory myelomas rarely occur.

## ■ Major Radiographic Features

1. Multiple small, discrete lesions are identifiable, involving one or several bones.
2. The tumor occasionally may present as a solitary osseous lesion.

3. The lesion is purely lytic.
4. The surrounding bone does not show a sclerotic reaction, nor is there periosteal reaction.
5. Endosteal scalloping may be identified.
6. Expansion of the affected bone and an associated soft tissue mass are common.

### ■ Radiographic Differential Diagnosis

1. Metastatic carcinoma.
2. Malignant lymphoma.
3. Fibrosarcoma.

### ■ Pathologic Features

#### Gross

1. The tumor tissue is generally soft and friable.
2. The color of the tissue varies from reddish to gray-white and grossly may appear similar to that of malignant lymphoma.
3. Extension into soft tissue may be discovered at the time of biopsy.

#### Microscopic

1. At low magnification the pattern is that of a cellular tumor lacking production of matrix.
2. The amount of cytoplasm on the cells varies but generally is abundant.
3. At higher magnification the nuclei generally are eccentrically placed in the cytoplasm and show a clumped chromatin pattern.
4. A cytoplasmic clearing adjacent to the nucleus (perinuclear hof) is frequently discernible.
5. Amyloid may be present as large masses of amorphous eosinophilic material. In such cases,

a foreign-body giant cell reaction may be elicited by the amyloid.
6. Mitotic activity is generally not brisk.

### ■ Pathologic Differential Diagnosis

Benign lesions:
1. Chronic osteomyelitis.
Malignant lesions:
1. Malignant lymphoma.

### ■ Treatment

**Primary Modality:** The mainstay of treatment is chemotherapy. Radiation therapy is effective in controlling localized lesions that are causing disabling pain or limitation of activity. The patient with solitary myeloma requires high-dose radiation for control of the disease.

**Other Possible Approaches:** surgical intervention with internal fixation of impending or actual pathologic fractures. Decompressive laminectomy may be indicated in patients with compressive myelopathy, and spinal stabilization is occasionally warranted.

### References

Bataille R, and Sany J: Solitary myeloma: clinical and prognostic features of a review of 114 cases. Cancer 48:845–851, 1981.

Kelly JJ Jr, Kyle RA, Miles JM, and Dyck PJ: Osteosclerotic myeloma and peripheral neuropathy. Neurology (NY) 33:202–210, 1983.

Kyle RA: Multiple myeloma: review of 869 cases. Mayo Clin Proc 50:29–40, 1975.

Kyle RA: Long-term survival in multiple myeloma. N Engl J Med 308:314–316, 1983.

Kyle RA, and Elveback LR: Management and prognosis of multiple myeloma. Mayo Clin Proc 51:751–760, 1976.

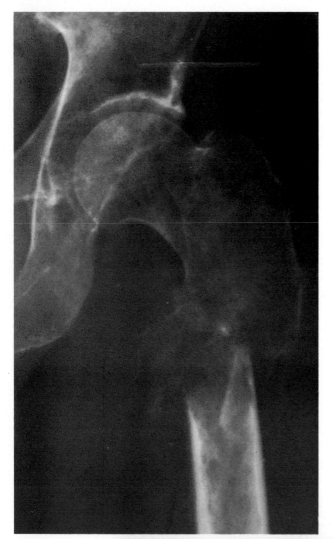

**Figure 25–1.** This radiograph illustrates a large, purely lytic lesion involving the proximal femur. The tumor has expanded the femur, resulting in pathologic fracture. The underlying process is myeloma.

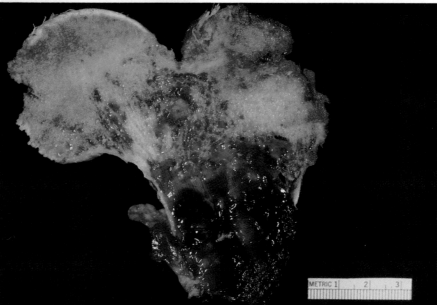

**Figure 25–2.** The gross pathologic features in this case correlate well with its radiographic features in Figure 25–1. Grossly myeloma is a soft, fish flesh–like lesion, as is shown here. Hemorrhage is commonly seen, in this case the result of the pathologic fracture that necessitated the resection of the proximal femur.

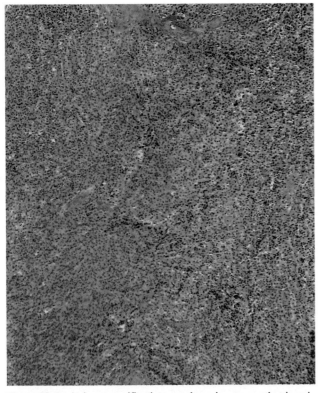

**Figure 25–3.** At low magnification, myeloma is a tumor that is uniform in appearance. The tumor is composed of round cells without any evidence of stromal proliferation.

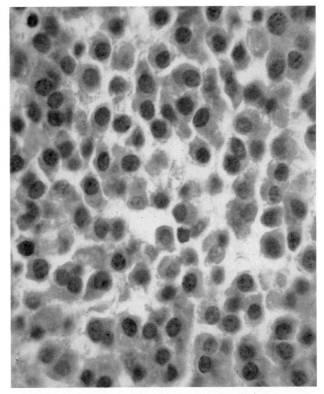

**Figure 25–5.** At high magnification, the proliferating plasma cells show abundant cytoplasm and an eccentrically located nucleus. Well-differentiated myelomas have cytologic features that deviate minimally from benign plasma cells; in such cases, chronic osteomyelitis may be included in the histologic differential diagnosis.

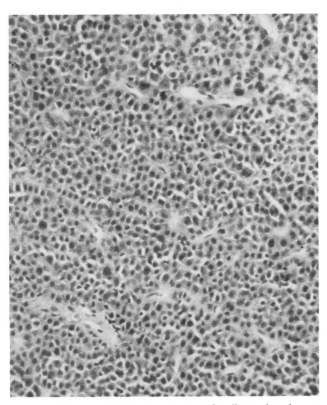

**Figure 25–4.** In contrast with most cases of malignant lymphoma, myeloma is generally composed of a homogeneous population of cells. This case illustrates such a proliferation of uniform cells.

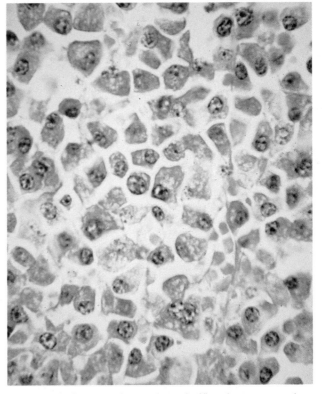

**Figure 25–6.** Some myelomas show significantly greater nuclear pleomorphism. In such cases the differential diagnosis will include immunoblastic lymphoma. However, some evidence of plasmacytic differentiation, as illustrated in this case, usually is seen.

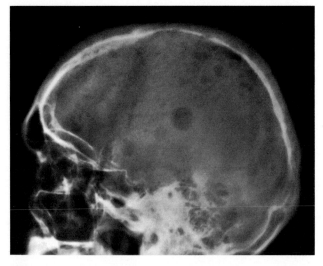

**Figure 25–7.** Multiple discrete lytic calvarial lesions, seen in this radiograph, are the hallmark of multiple myeloma.

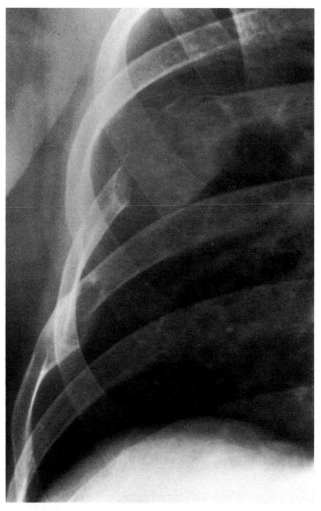

**Figure 25–9.** When myeloma involves the flat bone a soft tissue mass may be evident, as is shown in this example of myeloma involving two ribs.

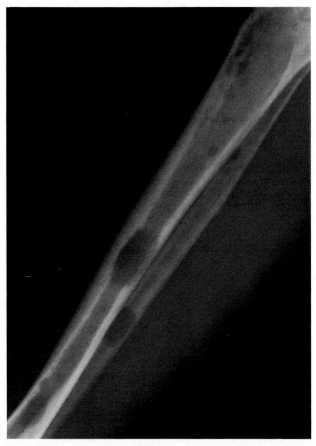

**Figure 25–8.** The long bone lesions of multiple myeloma show the same general radiographic features as do those of flat bones, as is shown in this radiograph illustrating tibial and fibular involvement.

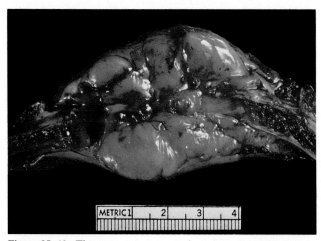

**Figure 25–10.** The gross appearance of myeloma is similar to malignant lymphoma, as is shown in this case involving the rib. Extension of the tumor into the soft tissues, as is seen in Figure 25–9, is present.

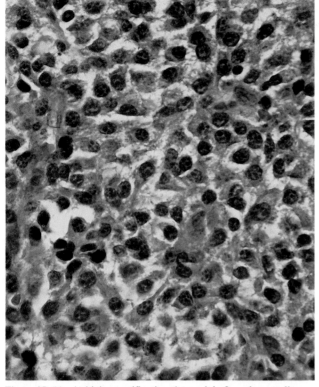

**Figure 25–11.** At high magnification the nuclei of myeloma cells are eccentrically placed and lie within abundant cytoplasm. A perinuclear clearing is frequently evident in the cytoplasm, as this photomicrograph illustrates.

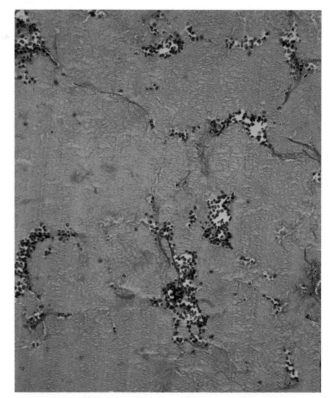

**Figure 25–13.** In some cases of myeloma, amyloid formation may be so prominent as to overwhelm the plasmacytic proliferation. Such is the case in this tumor involving the fourth thoracic vertebra.

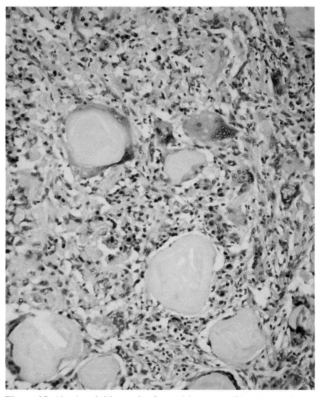

**Figure 25–12.** Amyloid may be formed in cases of myeloma. Such amyloid may result in a foreign body–type giant cell reaction, as shown in this photomicrograph.

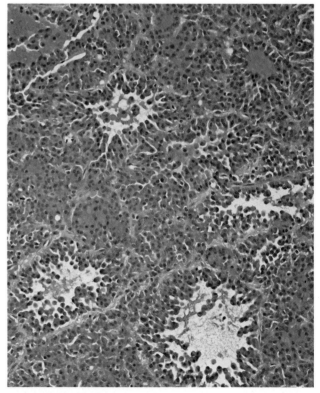

**Figure 25–14.** Myeloma grows in a noncohesive manner, and in some cases the resulting pattern may even resemble gland formation, as in metastatic adenocarcinoma. This case of myeloma shows such a pseudogland histologic pattern of growth.

# CHAPTER 26

# Mastocytosis (Mast Cell Disease)

*Peak age:*
Adulthood.
*Male to female ratio:*
Approximately 1 to 1.
*Most common location:*
May involve any bone and most commonly involves multiple bones.

## ■ Clinical Symptoms

1. Pigmented skin rash may be the patient's presenting complaint (urticaria pigmentosa).
2. Abdominal fullness may be experienced (hepatosplenomegaly).
3. Abdominal cramping and diarrhea may occur.
4. The lesion may be an incidental finding on x-ray and is usually mistaken for metastatic carcinoma.

## ■ Clinical Signs

1. The pigmented rash urticates when rubbed (urticaria pigmentosa).
2. Hepatosplenomegaly may be found on physical examination.

## ■ Major Radiographic Features

1. Skeletal involvement is most commonly diffuse; focal lesions are occasionally superimposed on diffuse disease, whereas focal lesions alone are unusual.
2. Diffuse osteopenia is the most common presentation, but diffuse sclerosis or mixed lysis and sclerosis are also seen.
3. Focal lesions are usually sclerotic or mixed.

## ■ Radiographic Differential Diagnosis

1. Osteoporosis.
2. Diffuse myeloma.
3. Lymphoma.

## ■ Pathologic Features

### Gross

1. Lesional tissue may be too ossified to cut with frozen section.

### Microscopic

1. At low magnification the bone shows diffuse permeation of the medullary space by a uniform population of small, regular cells. The cells are usually concentrated around bony trabeculae and are associated with fibrosis.
2. The trabeculae may show sclerosis, with increased thickness and greater irregularity than normal.
3. At higher magnification the cells are uniform, with a faintly granular cytoplasm.
4. The nuclei are regular, round to oval in shape, and have a finely stippled chromatin pattern.
5. The cells may show a tendency to spindle, and

in some areas the proliferation exhibits a granuloma-like quality.
6. Eosinophils may form a prominent part of the infiltrate.
7. Special stains may be used to demonstrate the metachromatic granules within the cytoplasm of the mast cells.

## ■ Pathologic Differential Diagnosis

Benign lesions:
1. Histiocytosis X.
2. Granulomatous osteomyelitis.
3. Nonspecific reactive changes.
Malignant lesions:
1. Hairy cell leukemia.
2. Malignant lymphoma.
3. Metastatic breast carcinoma.

## ■ Treatment

**Primary Modality:** depends upon the extent of disease. In children with limited disease the prognosis is good. In patients with skeletal involvement the prognosis is guarded but good. Rarely is there associated mast cell leukemia. Resection with a marginal or wide surgical margin is applicable for cases with limited disease.

**Other Possible Approaches:** chemotherapy.

## References

Barer M, Peterson LFA, Dahlin DC, et al: Mastocytosis with osseous lesions resembling metastatic malignant lesions in bone. J Bone Joint Surg 50A:142–152, 1968.
Havard CWH, and Scott RB: Urticaria pigmentosa with visceral and skeletal lesions. Q J Med 28:459–470, 1959.
Webb TA, Li CY, and Yam LT: Systemic mast cell disease: a clinical and hematopathologic study of 26 cases. Cancer 49:927–938, 1982.

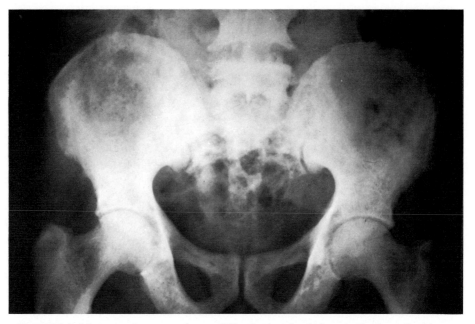

**Figure 26–1.** Mastocytosis may produce multifocal sclerosing lesions, as is shown in this case involving the pelvic bones. Such lesions are commonly mistaken for metastatic osteoblastic carcinoma.

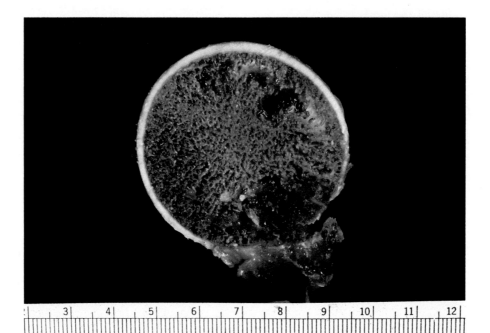

**Figure 26–2.** Grossly mastocytosis may be relatively inapparent. Although this femoral head showed diffuse involvement microscopically, only some thickening of the bony trabeculae was grossly evident.

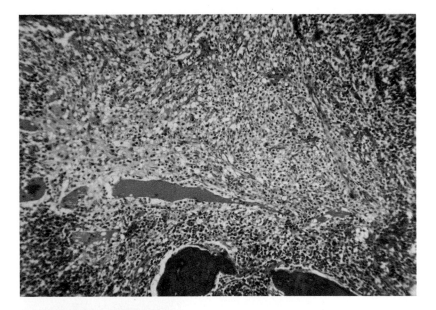

**Figure 26–3.** At low magnification the marrow space may show diffuse replacement in cases of mastocytosis. Even at this level of magnification the uniform cytologic features of the infiltrate are evident.

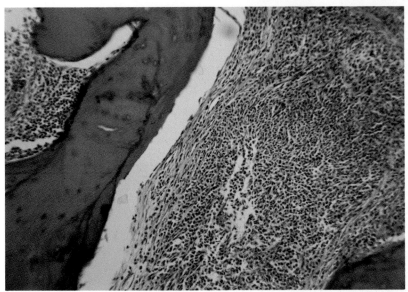

**Figure 26–4.** Fibrosis of the marrow space and bony sclerosis, as are evident in this case of mastocytosis involving the ilium, may also be seen.

**Figure 26–5.** Ultrastructurally mastocytosis is characterized by large cytoplasmic granules, as is illustrated in this sample of the lesion in a case involving the femoral head.

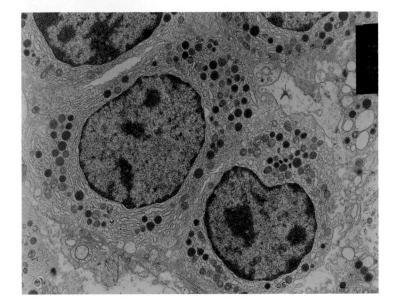

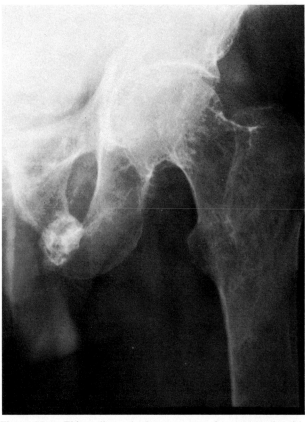

**Figure 26–6.** This radiograph shows a case of mastocytosis with diffuse skeletal demineralization and fracture of the pubic ramus.

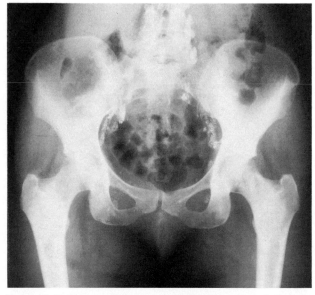

**Figure 26–7.** This case illustrates the diffuse bony sclerosis that may be seen in mastocytosis.

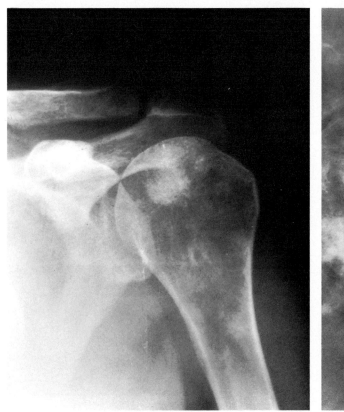

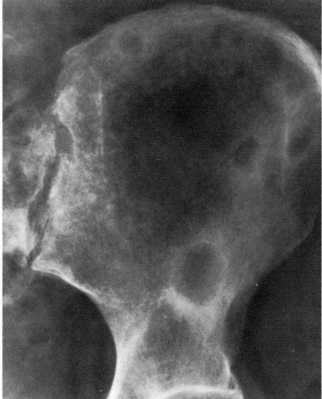

A

B

**Figure 26–8.** These radiographs show the shoulder (*A*) and pelvis (*B*) of a patient with mastocytosis. Some of the focal lesions are sclerotic; others are lytic, with surrounding sclerosis.

# SECTION ■ 5

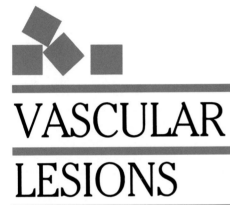

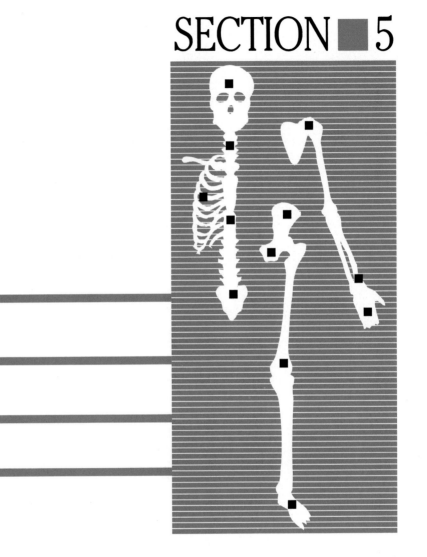

## VASCULAR
## LESIONS

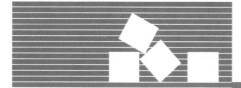

# CHAPTER 27

# Hemangioma

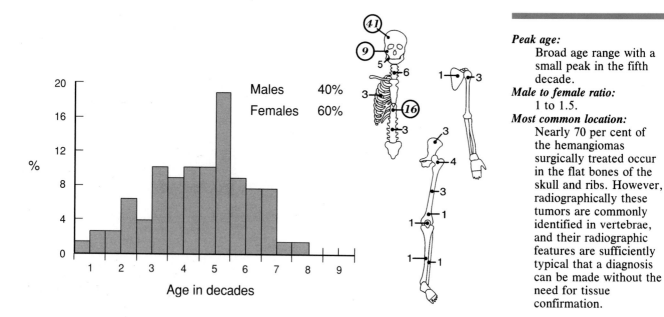

Males 40%
Females 60%

% 

Age in decades

**Peak age:**
Broad age range with a small peak in the fifth decade.
**Male to female ratio:**
1 to 1.5.
**Most common location:**
Nearly 70 per cent of the hemangiomas surgically treated occur in the flat bones of the skull and ribs. However, radiographically these tumors are commonly identified in vertebrae, and their radiographic features are sufficiently typical that a diagnosis can be made without the need for tissue confirmation.

■ **Clinical Symptoms**

1. The majority of hemangiomas are incidental findings on x-rays.
2. Swelling is frequently noted and is related to expansion of the affected bone. This is particularly true of lesions involving the skull.
3. Local pain is a less common complaint.
4. Spinal lesions may produce spinal cord compression.

■ **Clinical Signs**

1. Local pain and swelling are frequently seen in cases involving the skull and ribs.
2. Vertebral lesions may result in a compression fracture and resultant neurologic signs.
3. Severe hemorrhage may be encountered at the time of surgery.

■ **Major Radiographic Features**

1. In the calvarium:
   A. The lesion is small and oval with sharp margins.
   B. The lesion has a sunburst or granular appearance.
   C. 15 per cent are multicentric.

2. In the spine:
   A. The lesion has a "corduroy" or honeycombed appearance.
   B. It has a polka-dot appearance on computed tomography (CT) scan.
   C. The lesion may have a soft tissue mass or an associated pathologic fracture.

3. In the long bones: no specific appearance.

■ **Radiographic Differential Diagnosis**

1. For calvarial lesions:
   A. Histiocytosis X.
   B. Epidermoid cyst.
2. For vertebral lesions:
   A. Paget's disease.
   B. Metastatic carcinoma.
3. For long bone lesions:
   A. Hemangioendothelial sarcoma.
   B. Other sarcomas.

■ **Pathologic Features**

*Gross*

1. Grossly these lesions are soft, friable, red, and bloody.
2. Tumors may be more firm and fleshy if they are capillary in type.
3. Bony trabeculae may be grossly evident coursing through the tumor and are the counterpart of the "sunburst" seen radiographically in some cases.

*Microscopic*

1. At low magnification these lesions may show large, cavernous vascular spaces or small capillary-type vascular spaces.
2. The vascular nature is evident on low magnification, with the vascular spaces being lined by a thin, attenuated endothelial lining.
3. At higher magnification the endothelial cells are inconspicuous, as are their nuclei, which are small and dark.

■ **Pathologic Differential Diagnosis**

Benign lesions:
1. Disappearing bone disease.
2. Lymphangioma.
Malignant lesions:
1. Hemangioendothelial sarcoma.
2. Adamantinoma.

■ **Treatment**

**Primary Modality:** Observation is recommended for the usual lesion with an asymptomatic presentation. Curettage and grafting are utilized in the symptomatic lesion.

**Other Possible Approaches:** The symptomatic spinal lesion is treated with radiation therapy, with a dose of 3000 to 4000 rads. Surgical treatment with laminectomy is reserved for patients with spinal cord compression. Spinal angiography is helpful in these instances.

**References**

Asch MJ, Cohen AH, and Moore TC: Hepatic and splenic lymphangiomatosis with skeletal involvement: report of a case and review of the literature. Surgery 76:334–339, 1974.

Campanacci M, Cenni F, and Giunti A: Angectasie, amartomi, e neoplasmi vascolari dello scheletro ("angiomi," emangioendotelioma, emantiosarcoma). Chir Organi Mov 58:472–496, 1969.

Dorfman HD, Steiner GC, and Jeffe JL: Vascular tumors of bone. Hum Pathol 2:349–376, 1971.

Karlin CA, and Brower AC: Multiple primary hemangiomas of bone. AJR 129:162–164, 1977.

Unni KK, Ivins JC, Beabout JW, and Dahlin DC: Hemangioma, hemangiopericytoma, and hemangioendothelioma (angiosarcoma) of bone. Cancer 27:1403–1414, 1971.

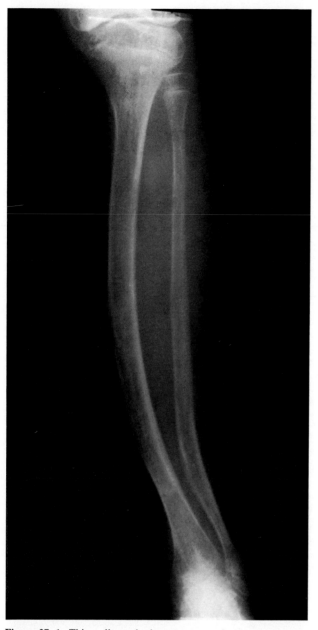

**Figure 27–1.** This radiograph shows an extensive hemangioma of the lower leg involving the soft tissues as well as the tibia and fibula. The bones contain lytic areas and are attenuated and bowed.

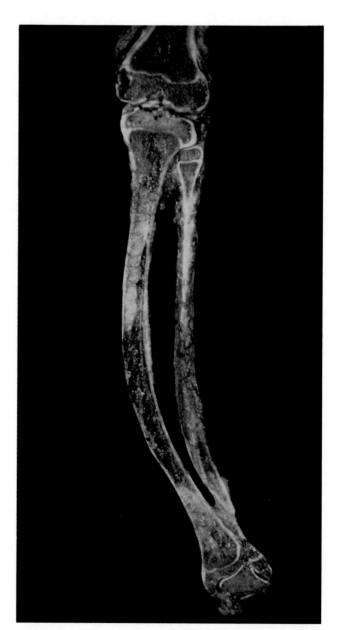

**Figure 27–2.** A gross specimen from the case shown in Figure 27–1 demonstrates the marked bowing of the tibia and fibula that was evident radiographically. Grossly hemangiomas are red, hemorrhagic lesions that may bleed extensively at the time of biopsy.

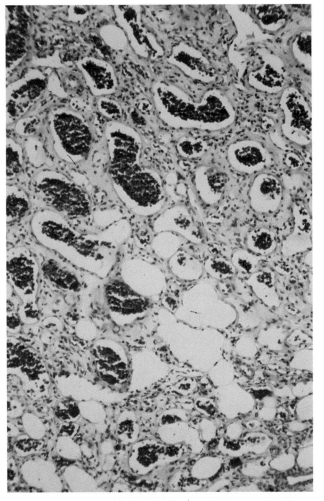

**Figure 27–3.** At low magnification hemangiomas may show large, dilated vascular spaces, as seen in this case. Such lesions are termed cavernous hemangiomas. In other cases small, capillary-like spaces may predominate; these lesions are termed capillary hemangiomas.

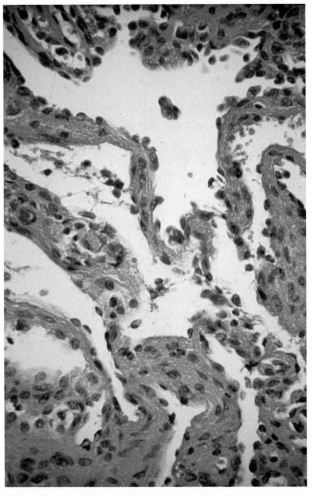

**Figure 27–4.** At high magnification, the endothelial cells lining the vascular spaces are inconspicuous. This feature helps to distinguish hemangiomas from low-grade hemangioendothelial sarcomas. The nuclei of the endothelial cells in a hemangioma are dark-staining and are flattened adjacent to the vascular lumina.

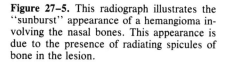

**Figure 27–5.** This radiograph illustrates the "sunburst" appearance of a hemangioma involving the nasal bones. This appearance is due to the presence of radiating spicules of bone in the lesion.

A                                                                                           B

**Figure 27–6.** The calvarium is a common location for hemangiomas. *A*, This radiograph illustrates a case with multicentric involvement showing three frontal bone lesions with sharp margination and a granular appearance. The gross appearance of such calvarial hemangiomas is shown in *B*. The radiating spicules of bone are visible traversing the lesion.

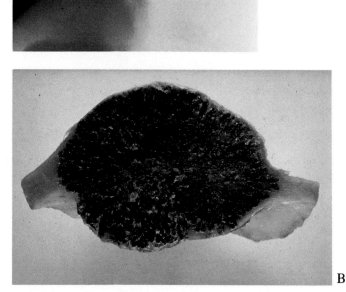

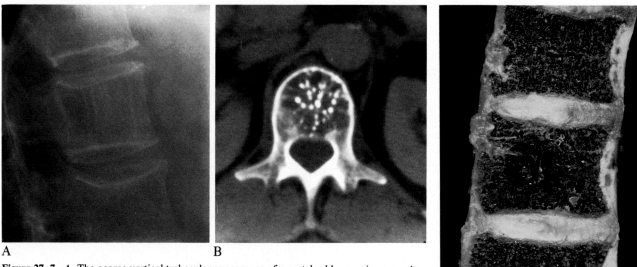

A                                           B

**Figure 27–7.** *A*, The coarse vertical trabecular appearance of a vertebral hemangioma results in the so-called corduroy vertebra. *B* shows the CT cross-sectional appearance of a similar vertebral hemangioma. In cross-section the coarse trabeculae result in a polka-dot pattern.

**Figure 27–8.** Grossly, hemangiomas of the vertebrae are common findings during post mortem examination, as shown in this photograph. Such lesions are small and generally clinically silent.

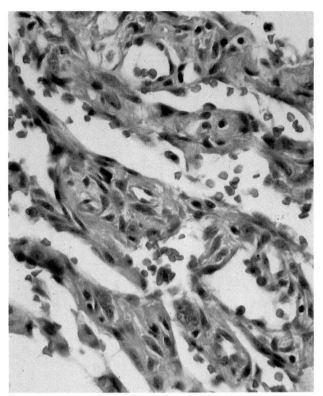

**Figure 27–10.** The histologic features of phantom bone disease are often indistinguishable from a hemangioma, as this example of a femoral lesion demonstrates. The clinical history is often helpful in separating these two conditions.

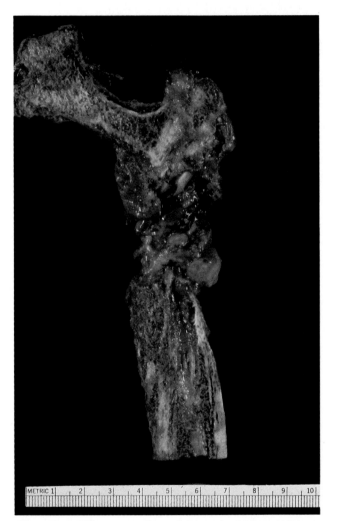

**Figure 27–9.** This gross specimen of the proximal femur exhibits the bony dissolution associated with phantom bone disease (massive osteolysis, Gorham's disease).

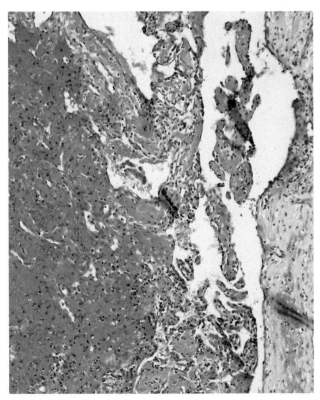

**Figure 27–11.** Other benign vascular processes may involve the bone and show a histologic pattern similar to a hemangioma. This photomicrograph shows an example of an arteriovenous fistula with associated thrombus formation that resulted in a distal fibular defect.

# CHAPTER 28

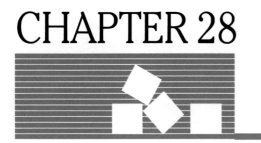

# Hemangioendothelial Sarcoma (Hemangioendothelioma, Epithelioid Hemangioendothelioma, Histiocytoid Hemangioma, and Angiosarcoma)

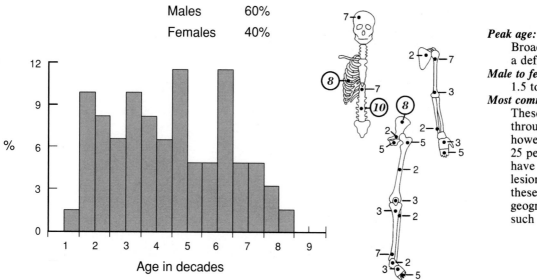

Males 60%
Females 40%

Age in decades

*Peak age:*
    Broad age range without a definite peak.
*Male to female ratio:*
    1.5 to 1.
*Most common location:*
    These tumors occur throughout the skeleton; however, approximately 25 per cent of cases have multiple osseous lesions. About half of these occur in one geographic location, such as a limb.

■ **Clinical Symptoms**

1. Pain is the usual clinical symptom.
2. Rarely a mass may be noted if the lesion involves a superficial bone.

■ **Clinical Signs**

1. Local tenderness may be the only finding on physical examination.

■ **Major Radiographic Features**

1. There is no specific radiographic appearance.

2. The most common pattern is that of a purely lytic lesion without periosteal reaction.
3. The radiographic appearance correlates with the histologic grade. High-grade lesions appear more permeative and destructive than do low-grade lesions.
4. Multifocal disease may be seen and, when present, frequently tends to cluster in one anatomic region.

■ **Radiographic Differential Diagnosis**

1. Osteosarcoma.

168

2. Fibrosarcoma.
3. Malignant fibrous histiocytoma.
4. Malignant lymphoma.
5. Metastatic carcinoma.
6. Hemangioma.

## ■ Pathologic Features

### Gross

1. The lesional tissue is usually grossly red and bloody.
2. Tumors vary in consistency but are generally soft. Residual bony trabeculae may be present, particularly in low-grade lesions, giving the tumor a firmer consistency.
3. Necrotic tumor may be present but is most often seen in high-grade lesions.

### Microscopic

1. The histologic features vary considerably in this group from low-grade tumors, which are obviously vasoformative, to high-grade, which may show areas of spindle cell proliferation without obvious vessel formation.
2. Low-grade tumors show plump endothelial cells lining vascular spaces. The nuclei on higher magnification may appear histiocytoid or epithelioid.
3. High-grade tumors show greater cytologic variation and mitotic activity and less histologic differentiation than their low-grade counterparts.
4. Reticulin stains may be helpful in defining the vascular nature of the tumor by showing that the proliferating cells are clustered within a meshwork of reticulin fibers.
5. Immunohistochemical stains for endothelial and mesenchymal markers (e.g., Factor VIII–related antigen and vimentin) are variably positive.

## ■ Pathologic Differential Diagnosis

Benign lesions:

1. Hemangioma.
2. Disappearing bone disease.

Malignant lesions:

1. Metastatic carcinoma.
2. Fibrosarcoma.
3. Telangiectatic osteosarcoma.
4. Adamantinoma.

## ■ Treatment

**Primary Modality:** Treatment is dependent on the grade of the lesion. Low-grade lesions that are unifocal may be treated with en bloc resection with a wide surgical margin. Low-grade multifocal lesions may be effectively treated with radiation therapy or amputation. High-grade lesions may be treated with either radiation therapy or ablative surgery, although some lesions are amenable to limb-saving resection.

**Other Possible Approaches:** Chemotherapy has been used with limited success in some cases of high-grade tumors.

## References

Campanacci M, Boriani S, and Giunti A: Hemangioendothelioma of bone: a study of 29 cases. Cancer 46:804–814, 1980.

Dorfman HD, Steiner GC, and Jaffe HL: Vascular tumors of bone. Hum Pathol 2:349–376, 1971.

Garcia-Moral CA: Malignant hemangioendothelioma of bone: review of world literature and report of two cases. Clin Orthop 82:70–79, 1972.

Rosai J, Gold J, and Landy R: The histiocytoid hemangiomas: a unifying concept embracing several previously described entities of skin, soft tissue, large vessels, bone and heart. Hum Pathol 10:707–730, 1979.

Unni KK, Ivins JC, Beabout JW, and Dahlin DC: Hemangioma, hemangiopericytoma, and hemangioendothelioma (angiosarcoma) of bone. Cancer 27:1403–1414, 1971.

Volpe R, and Mazabraud A: Hemangioendothelioma (angiosarcoma) of bone: a distinct pathologic entity with an unpredictable course. Cancer 49:727–736, 1981.

Weiss SW, and Enzinger FM: Epithelioid hemangioendothelioma: a vascular tumor often mistaken for a carcinoma. Cancer 50:970–981, 1982.

Wold LE, Unni KK, Beabout JW, et al: Hemangioendothelial sarcoma of bone. Am J Surg Pathol 6:59–70, 1982.

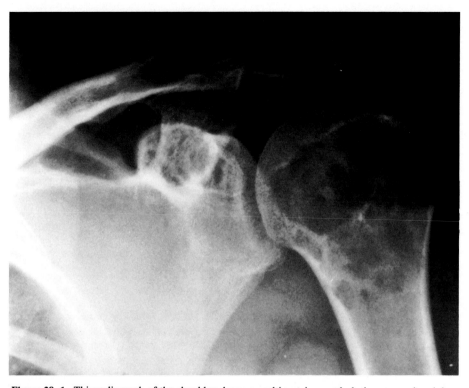

**Figure 28–1.** This radiograph of the shoulder shows a multicentric, purely lytic process involving the clavicle, scapula, and humerus. The presence of multiple lesions, generally purely lytic in character, in the same anatomic region suggests a diagnosis of hemangioendothelial sarcoma.

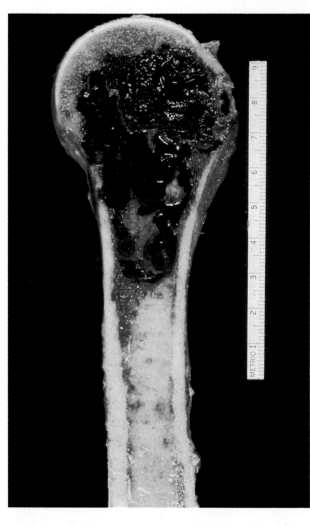

**Figure 28–2.** The gross specimen in this case of multicentric hemangioendothelial sarcoma correlates well with its radiographic appearance. These tumors generally are red and hemorrhagic. Although the tumor has not extended into the adjacent soft tissue, cortical erosion is evident.

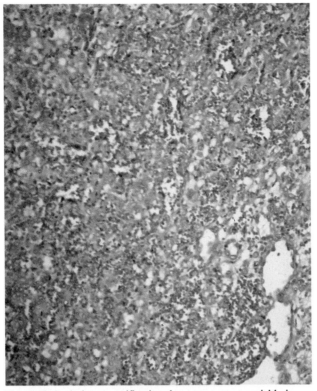

**Figure 28–3.** At low magnification these tumors are variable in appearance; in general, however, their vasoformative nature is evident. Most commonly the vascular spaces are small, as is demonstrated in this lesion from the humerus. (This is the same case as shown in Figures 28–1 and 28–2.)

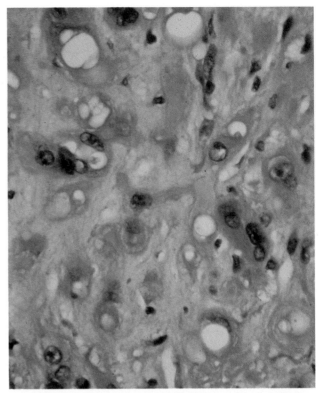

**Figure 28–5.** Grade 1 tumors, epithelioid hemangioendotheliomas, frequently contain a collagenized, chondroid-appearing stroma, as is shown in this photomicrograph. Also visible are cells with intracytoplasmic lumina.

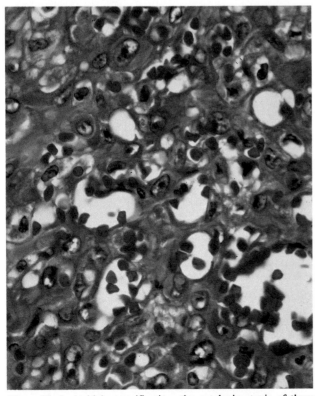

**Figure 28–4.** At high magnification, the cytologic atypia of these lesions varies from case to case. As this photomicrograph shows, the nuclei are plump, hyperchromatic, and variable in shape. They bulge into the vascular lumina, and tufting may occasionally be seen.

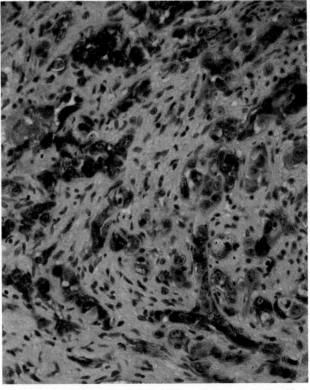

**Figure 28–6.** Markers of endothelial differentiation may be identified using immunohistochemical or ultrastructural analysis. This photomicrograph illustrates positive staining for Factor VIII–related antigen in a low-grade hemangioendothelial sarcoma.

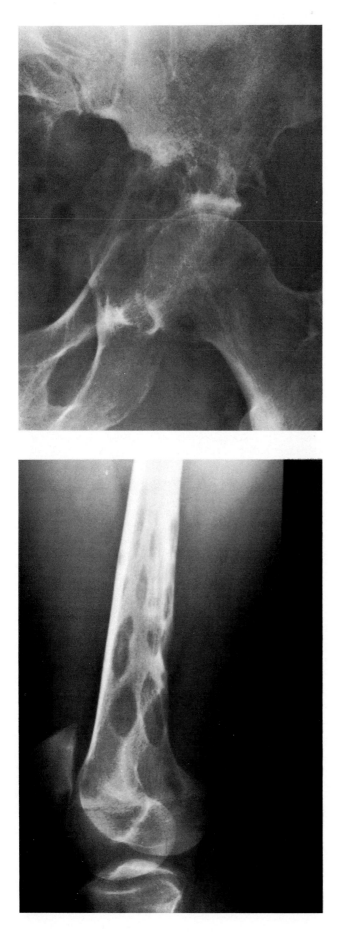

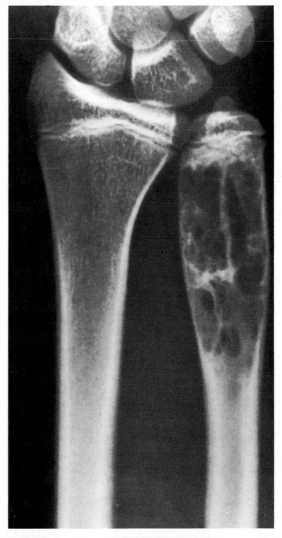

**Figure 28–7.** This radiograph illustrates the poorly marginated, lytic appearance of a hemangioendothelial sarcoma involving the acetabulum. The radiographic appearance suggests malignancy but is otherwise nonspecific.

**Figure 28–8.** An expansile lytic lesion in the distal ulnar metaphysis is shown in this radiograph. Low-grade hemangioendothelial sarcomas often have a benign radiographic appearance.

**Figure 28–9.** This radiograph shows an aggressive, lytic, multicentric process in the distal femur. High-grade hemangioendothelial sarcomas generally show this aggressive pattern of growth.

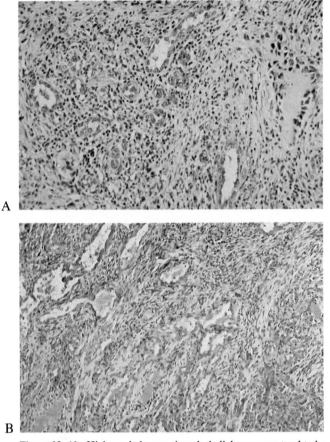

A

B

**Figure 28–10.** High-grade hemangioendothelial sarcomas tend to be less vasoformative, as the photomicrograph in *A* shows. In such cases a careful search must be made to identify the endothelial nature of the tumor. Although another lesion may be quite vasoformative (*B*), the gland-like appearance of such a lesion may suggest the diagnosis of metastatic adenocarcinoma.

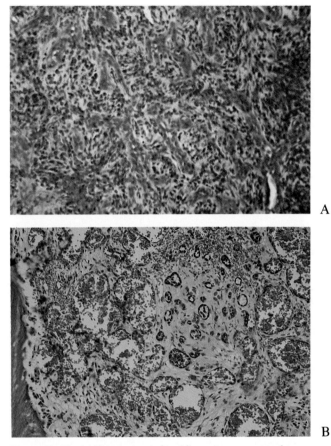

A

B

**Figure 28–11.** *A*, Numerous eosinophils may accompany hemangioendothelial sarcomas, whether they are low- or high-grade. This feature, when taken out of context, may suggest a diagnosis of eosinophilic granuloma. *B*, Other lesions may simulate the appearance of adamantinoma. The location of the lesion is helpful in distinguishing between these two conditions.

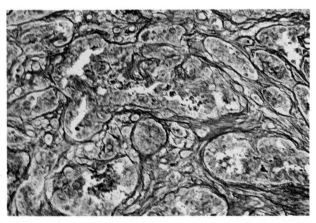

**Figure 28–12.** Special stains may help to show the clustered pattern of growth that is present in hemangioendothelial sarcomas. This reticulin stain highlights this histologic feature, which may not be obvious in high-grade tumors with hematoxylin and eosin–stained sections.

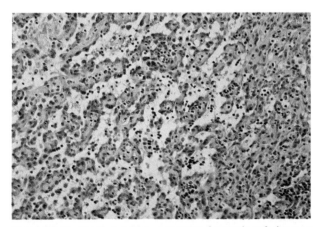

**Figure 28–13.** Papillary tufting, a common feature in soft tissue angiosarcomas, is uncommon in bony lesions. This case of a femoral lesion in a patient with multicentric disease demonstrates this histologic feature.

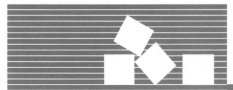

# CHAPTER 29

# Hemangiopericytoma

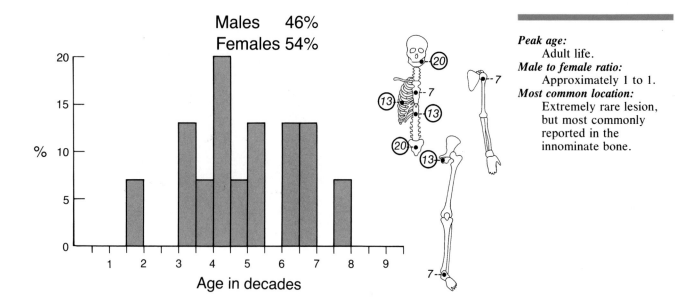

Males 46%
Females 54%

% (y-axis), Age in decades (x-axis)

*Peak age:*
Adult life.
*Male to female ratio:*
Approximately 1 to 1.
*Most common location:*
Extremely rare lesion, but most commonly reported in the innominate bone.

■ **Clinical Symptoms**

1. Local pain is present.
2. Swelling is noted in the region of the tumor.

■ **Clinical Signs**

1. A mass lesion is palpable on physical examination.
2. The mass most commonly is tender to palpation.

■ **Major Radiographic Features**

1. This rare primary tumor of bone generally has a nonspecific radiographic appearance.
2. Over two-thirds are purely lytic.
3. Most have a malignant appearance, and their radiographic appearance roughly correlates with the histologic grade of the tumor.
4. A honeycombed appearance occasionally is seen.

■ **Radiographic Differential Diagnosis**

1. Any lytic primary bone tumor.
2. Lytic metastatic tumors of bone.

■ **Pathologic Features**

*Gross*

1. The tumor is usually firm in consistency.
2. The lesional tissue is most often red and bloody.

*Microscopic*

1. At low magnification this tumor is composed of round to oval cells.
2. The tumor is hypercellular.
3. Numerous thin-walled blood vessels course through the tumor.
4. The blood vessels are branched and "staghorn" in shape.

5. At higher magnification the degree of cytologic atypia is variable.
6. Mitotic activity in the tumor is also variable.
7. No matrix is produced by the tumor cells.

## ■ Pathologic Differential Diagnosis

Benign lesions:
1. Glomus tumor.
2. Capillary hemangioma.

Malignant lesions:
1. Mesenchymal chondrosarcoma.
2. Small cell osteosarcoma.
3. Metastatic hemangiopericytoma (particularly common with hemangiopericytomas of the meninges).

## ■ Treatment

**Primary Modality:** en bloc resection with a wide margin and skeletal reconstruction if feasible. Amputation may be necessary to achieve an adequately wide margin.

**Other Possible Approaches:** radiotherapy for surgically inaccessible lesions. Multiple-drug chemotherapy protocols used in an adjuvant setting may be employed.

## References

Dunlop J: Primary haemangiopericytoma of bone: report of two cases. J Bone Joint Surg 55B:854–857, 1973.
Wold LW, Unni KK, Cooper KL, et al: Hemangiopericytoma of bone. Am J Surg Pathol 6:53–58, 1982.

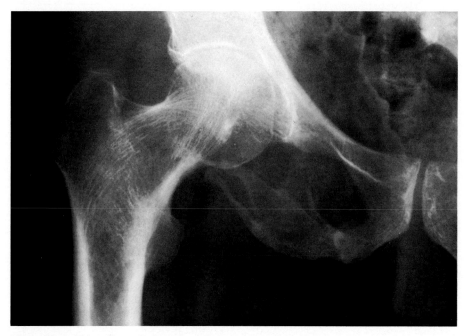

**Figure 29–1.** This radiograph shows a purely lytic hemangiopericytoma of the ischium. The lesion exhibits features of a malignant lesion but is otherwise nonspecific.

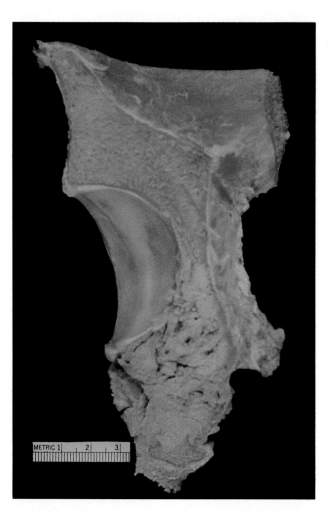

**Figure 29–2.** Grossly the ischial hemangiopericytoma is relatively nondescript. The lesional tissue is firm and fibrous in consistency. Such tissue may be reddish and bloody.

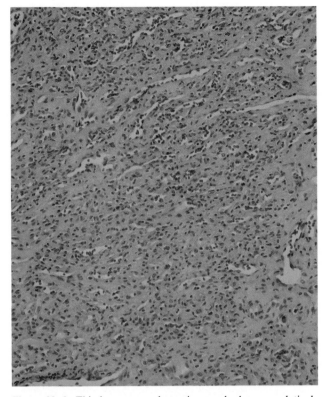

**Figure 29–3.** This low-power photomicrograph shows a relatively hypocellular tumor composed of ovoid cells arranged around vascular spaces. This tumor of the thoracic vertebra in a 38-year-old male exhibits histologic features of a ''benign'' hemangiopericytoma.

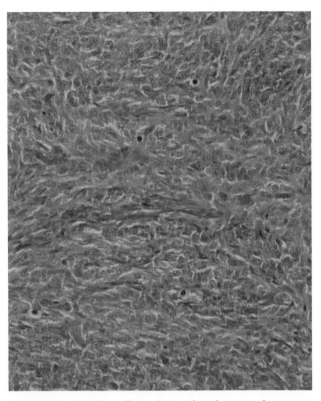

**Figure 29–5.** Frankly malignant hemangiopericytomas show greater cellular pleomorphism and atypia, as can be seen in this photomicrograph of a primary osseous tumor that also shows moderate mitotic activity.

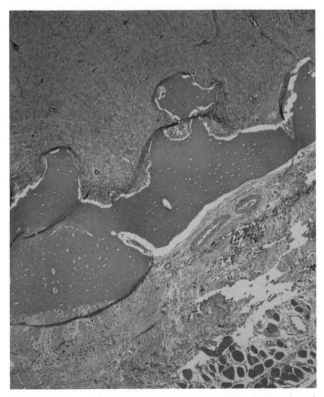

**Figure 29–4.** At low magnification more aggressive hemangiopericytomas may show cortical erosion, as is evident in this lesion involving a rib.

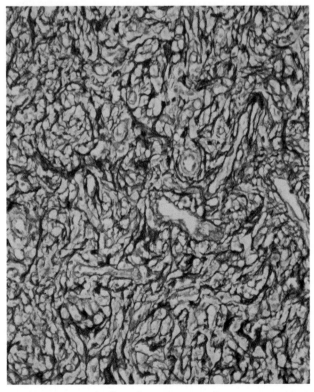

**Figure 29–6.** A reticulin stain, such as seen here, may accentuate the vascular nature of these tumors. The fine reticulin meshwork that surrounds each cell is helpful in identifying the lesion as a hemangiopericytoma.

**Figure 29–7.** A radiograph (*A*) and an axial MRI (*B*) of a hemangiopericytoma of the posterior lower femur show destruction of the cortex and extension into the soft tissues. The appearance favors malignancy. The lesion is seen best on MRI.

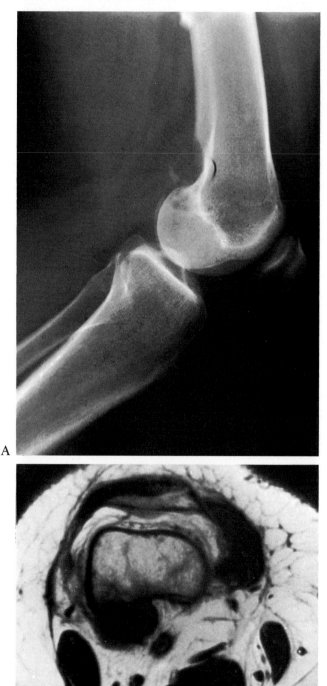

A

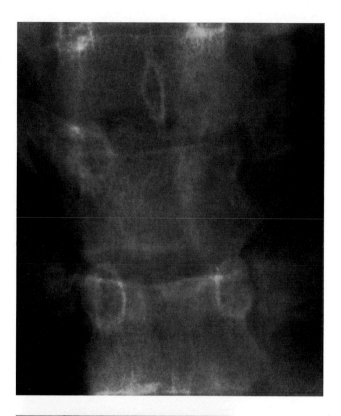

B

**Figure 29–8.** Hemangiopericytomas of the meninges show a propensity to osseous metastases, as can be seen in this radiograph of the thoracic spine. Note the lytic destruction of the left pedicle and adjacent vertebral body.

**Figure 29–9.** Glomus tumors are benign examples of pericytic tumors. These lesions are most commonly identified in the distal phalanx radiographically. Note the well-circumscribed lytic defect of the distal phalangeal tuft in this case.

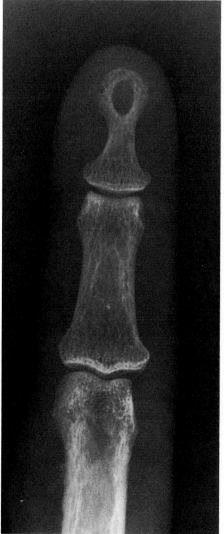

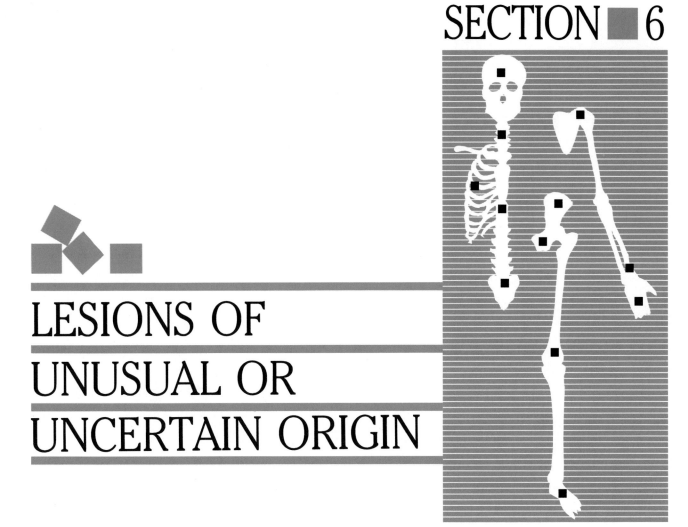

# SECTION ■ 6

# LESIONS OF UNUSUAL OR UNCERTAIN ORIGIN

# CHAPTER 30

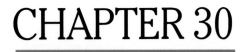

# Histiocytosis X (Langerhans' Cell Granulomatosis)

Males     62%
Females 38%

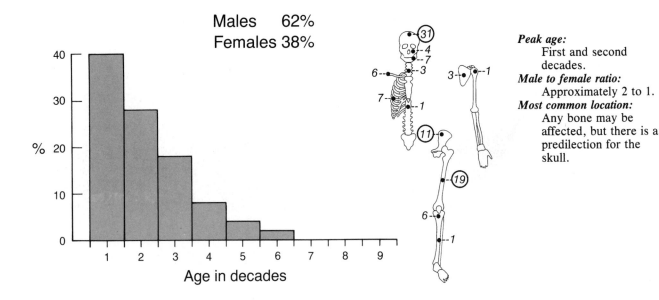

% 

Age in decades

**Peak age:**
First and second decades.
**Male to female ratio:**
Approximately 2 to 1.
**Most common location:**
Any bone may be affected, but there is a predilection for the skull.

■ **Clinical Symptoms**

1. Pain is the most frequent presenting complaint.
2. A swelling may also be noted in the region of the bone involved.
3. Only rarely will the lesion be discovered incidentally on radiographic examination.
4. Protean clinical symptoms are seen in multisystem disease, e.g., Hand-Schüller-Christian or Letterer-Siwe variants.
5. The patient may present with otorrhea.
6. Loose teeth may be the presenting complaint in patients with maxillary or mandibular involvement.
7. Excessive thirst may be a manifestation of associated central nervous system disease.

■ **Clinical Signs**

1. A mass may be palpable on physical examination.
2. Cutaneous seborrhea-like lesions may be identified, indicating skin involvement.
3. Hearing loss or decreased balance may indicate involvement of the mastoid region.
4. Marked tenderness in the region of the affected bone may be found on physical examination.

■ **Major Radiographic Features**

1. The radiographic appearance is highly variable; lesions tend to occur in flat bones, especially the calvarium.

2. Lesions range from solitary to innumerable.
3. Most lesions are lytic, with well-defined margins.
4. Expansion, solid periosteal new bone formation, and surrounding sclerosis may occur.
5. Lesions are often medullary and have an irregular or scalloped margin.
6. Many lesions have a double contour.
7. Spine involvement usually affects the vertebral body and results in uniform compression.
8. Other favored sites include the ribs, the clavicle, the neck of the scapula, and the supra-acetabular iliac bone.

■ **Radiographic Differential Diagnosis**

1. Osteomyelitis.
2. Primary osseous malignancies.
3. Metastases.

■ **Pathologic Features**

*Gross*

1. Lesional tissue is usually soft and may be "runny."
2. The tissue varies in color from gray-tan to pale red or yellow. The eosinophils may impart a greenish hue to the lesional tissue.
3. Pathologic fracture may be identified in resected specimens.

*Microscopic*

1. At low magnification the lesional tissue is arranged in a loose fashion. Necrosis is common.
2. The lesion is polymorphous, being composed of a variety of inflammatory cells including polymorphonuclear leukocytes, lymphocytes, plasma cells, multinucleated giant cells, and the characteristic Langerhans' histiocytes.
3. The Langerhans' cells are arranged in relatively solid sheets or clusters.

4. At higher magnification the characteristic cytologic features of the Langerhans' cell include:
   A. An indented or folded nucleus.
   B. A crisp nuclear membrane.
   C. A finely stippled chromatin pattern.
   D. Small, inconspicuous nucleoli.
   E. Abundant pale eosinophilic cytoplasm.
5. Eosinophils may be quite abundant; they may be clustered into small eosinophilic "abscesses."
6. Mitotic activity may be focally brisk.

■ **Pathologic Differential Diagnosis:**
Benign lesions:
   1. Osteomyelitis.
   2. Erdheim-Chester disease.
Malignant lesions:
   1. Malignant lymphoma.
   2. Malignant fibrous histiocytoma, inflammatory variant.

■ **Treatment**

**Primary Modality:** surgery or radiation therapy, usually radiation in low doses. A simple solitary lesion compromising the structural integrity of the bone is managed by curettage and bone grafting when surgically accessible.

**Other Possible Approaches:** With multiple lesions, a period of observation for patients with asymptomatic lesions may permit spontaneous healing. Direct injection of methylprednisolone acetate into the lesion has obtained encouraging results. For Hand-Schüller-Christian disease and Letterer-Siwe disease, corticosteroids and chemotherapy may be utilized.

**References**

Enriquez P, Dahlin DC, Hayles AB, and Henderson ED: Histiocytosis X: a clinical study. Mayo Clin Proc 42:88–99, 1967.
Wester SM, Beabout JW, Unni KK, and Dahlin DC: Langerhans' cell granulomatosis (histiocytosis X) of bone in adults. Am J Surg Pathol 6:413–426, 1982.

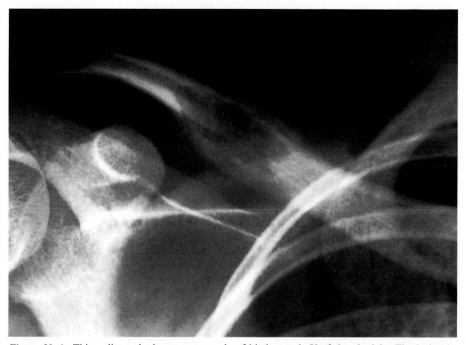

**Figure 30–1.** This radiograph shows an example of histiocytosis X of the clavicle. The lesion is poorly marginated, and associated new bone formation is present. A similar appearance could be caused by Ewing's sarcoma or osteomyelitis.

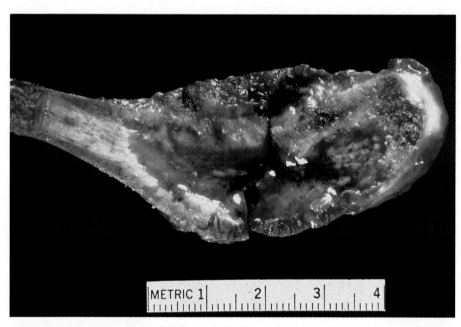

**Figure 30–2.** Another example of histiocytosis X of the clavicle demonstrates the gross pathologic features of the condition. The lesional tissue may be quite loose and runny. Lesions that extend beyond the cortex, as shown here, may simulate the appearance of a malignant neoplasm radiographically.

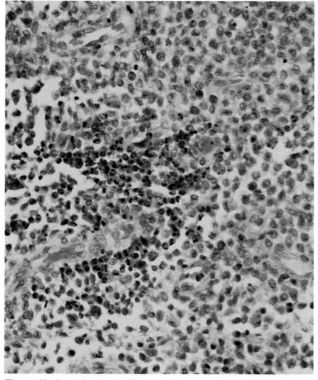

**Figure 30–3.** At low magnification histiocytosis X is a lesion composed of multiple cell types. Eosinophils may be prominent, as in this case, or sparse. In this lesion the loose nature of the process is evident, and an eosinophilic "abscess" is present.

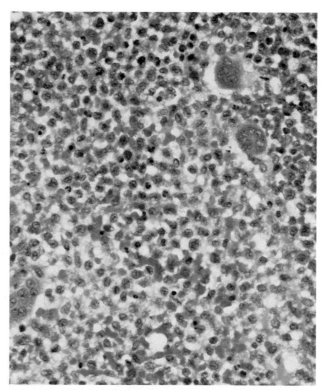

**Figure 30–5.** Multinucleated giant cells, as are shown in this photomicrograph, may be seen in histiocytosis X. Mitotic activity may be fairly brisk, but this feature does not appear to correlate with the clinical course of the disease.

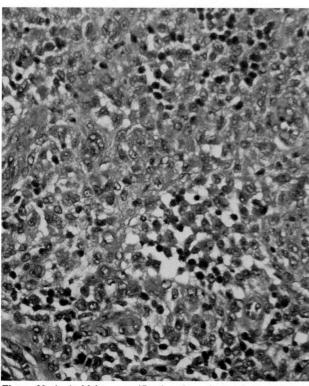

**Figure 30–4.** At higher magnification the polymorphous nature of the process is evident. The Langerhans'-type histiocytes have abundant cytoplasm and a coffee bean–shaped nucleus. Lymphocytes, plasma cells, and polymorphonuclear leukocytes are scattered through the lesional tissue.

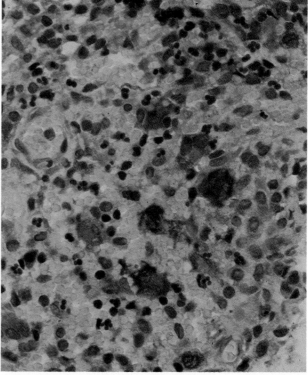

**Figure 30–6.** Immunohistochemical techniques may be helpful in substantiating the diagnosis of histiocytosis X. The polymorphous nature of the infiltrate frequently raises the differential diagnosis of chronic osteomyelitis. In such cases, immunostains for S-100 protein may be helpful in identifying the characteristic Langerhans' cells of histiocytosis X.

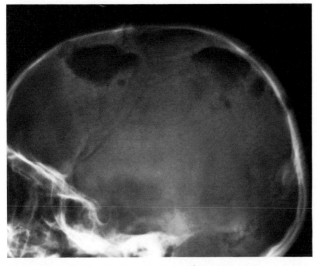

**Figure 30–7.** This radiograph shows multiple calvarial lesions, most of which are serpiginous with sharp margination. This is one of the radiographic appearances of histiocytosis X.

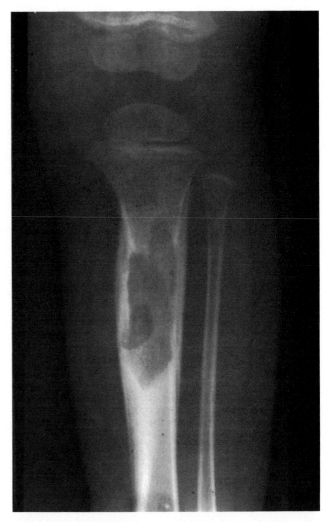

**Figure 30–9.** This radiograph demonstrates the typical appearance of histiocytosis X involving the tibial diaphysis. The medullary lesion has a serpiginous margin that is well defined. The "hole within a hole" appearance and the thick, solid periosteal new bone formation are also characteristic.

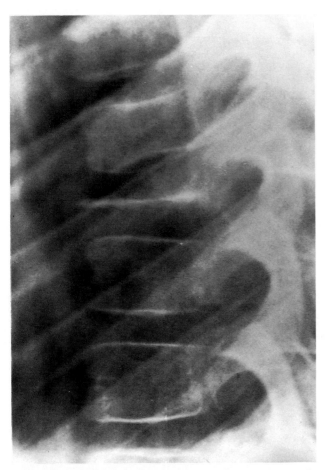

**Figure 30–8.** Uniform compression of a thoracic vertebra is shown in this radiograph. This condition, termed vertebra plana, is another presentation of histiocytosis X.

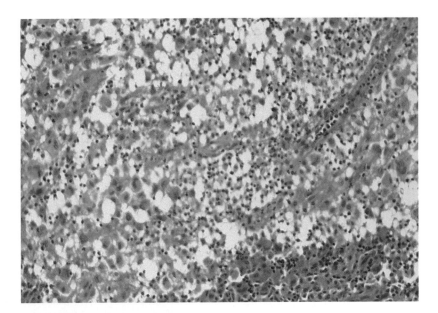

**Figure 30–10.** At low magnification lesional tissue in histiocytosis X often has a loose, edematous appearance, as is shown in this case of an L4 vertebral lesion.

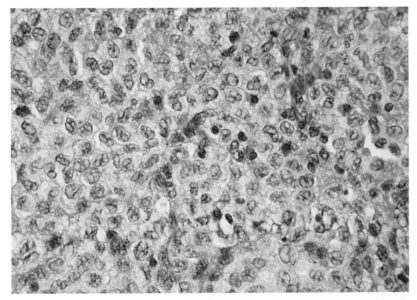

**Figure 30–11.** At high magnification the cytologic features of the nuclei of the Langerhans' cells are identifiable. The nucleus is oval or bean-shaped and has a characteristic longitudinal groove if viewed en face.

**Figure 30–12.** Ultrastructural investigation can help in identifying the characteristic features of histiocytosis X. The lobulated nucleus is identifiable (*A*), but the feature that is diagnostic of the condition is the presence of the characteristic granules (*B*).

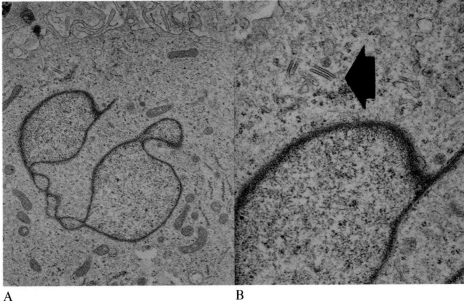

A                                    B

# CHAPTER 31

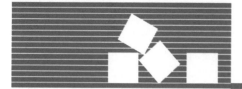

# Neurilemmoma

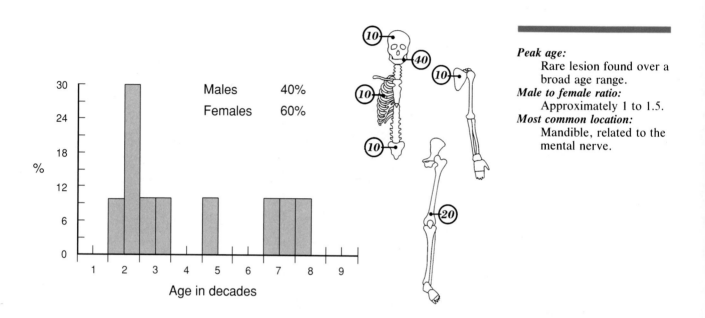

Males 40%
Females 60%

*Peak age:*
    Rare lesion found over a broad age range.
*Male to female ratio:*
    Approximately 1 to 1.5.
*Most common location:*
    Mandible, related to the mental nerve.

■ **Clinical Symptoms**

1. Many neurilemmomas are asymptomatic.
2. A minority of lesions produce pain.
3. A minority of lesions produce a swelling that is noticed by the patient.

■ **Clinical Signs**

1. There are generally no specific findings on physical examination.
2. A small mass lesion may be found if the lesion involves a superficial bone, e.g., the mandible.
3. Stigmata of neurofibromatosis may be present in some cases.

■ **Major Radiographic Features**

1. The lesion has a benign appearance, with sharp margins and a sclerotic rim.

2. Intraosseous tumors usually arise near the end of the bone and within the shaft.
3. Erosion of the bone by a tumor arising in nerves contiguous to bone is the most common presentation.

■ **Radiographic Differential Diagnosis**

1. Fibroma.
2. Fibrous dysplasia.
3. Chondromyxoid fibroma.
4. Neurofibroma.

■ **Pathologic Features**

*Gross*

1. The lesion is generally well circumscribed.
2. The tissue is firm in consistency but may show regions of myxoid and cystic change.

3. The tissue is yellow to brown in color.
4. The lesion's relationship to a nerve or its canal may be appreciated.

*Microscopic*

1. At low magnification the lesion is hypocellular and composed of spindle cells.
2. Between the spindle cells is a loose, myxoid-appearing matrix.
3. Focally the nuclei of the spindle cells may be clustered in a linear fashion (Verocay bodies).
4. At higher magnification the nuclei are generally small and hyperchromic. However, they may become irregular in size, shape, and staining characteristics—features that are ascribed to degeneration.
5. No mitotic figures are identified.

## ■ Pathologic Differential Diagnosis

Benign lesions:
1. Myxoma.

Malignant lesions:
1. Fibrosarcoma.
2. Malignant fibrous histiocytoma, myxoid variant.

## ■ Treatment

**Primary Modality:** conservative surgical excision with a marginal margin.

**Other Possible Approaches:** These lesions, which may become very large when they arise in the sacrum, can be "shelled out," preserving sacral nerve roots.

## References

Fawcett KJ, and Dahlin DC: Neurilemmoma of bone. Am J Clin Pathol 47:759–766, 1967.

Gordon EJ: Solitary intraosseous neurilemmoma of the tibia: review of intraosseous neurilemmoma and neurofibroma. Clin Orthop 117:271–282, 1976.

Vicas E, Bourdua S, and Charest F: Le neurilemmome du sacrum: presentation d'un cas. Union Med Can 103:1057–1060, 1974.

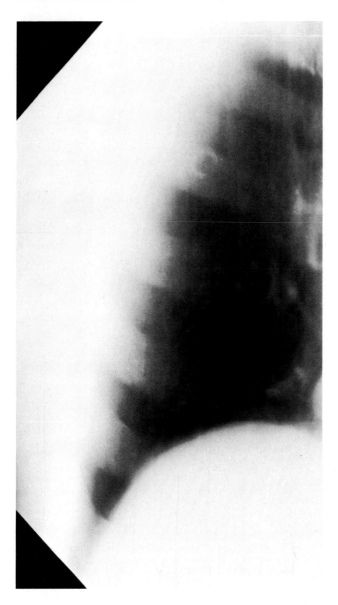

**Figure 31–1.** This radiograph shows a small oval neurilemmoma of the anterior rib. The sharp margination, sclerotic rim, and cortical expansion indicate a benign process.

**Figure 31–2.** This resected rib (also seen in Fig. 31–1) shows cystic degenerative changes. Such changes frequently occur in neurilemmomas but may also be found in fibrous dysplasia involving the rib.

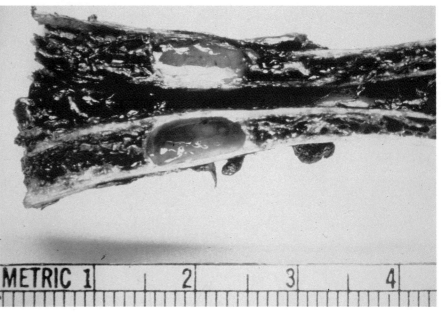

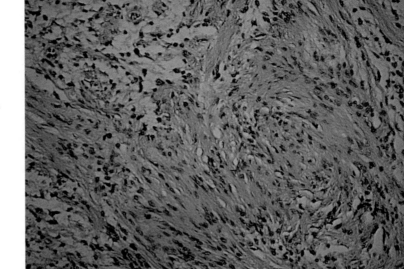

**Figure 31–3.** This photomicrograph of a mandibular neurilemmoma shows the admixture of spindle and round cells commonly seen in this lesion. Frequently lipid-laden histiocytes are so prominent as to be evident as yellowish areas in the tumor grossly.

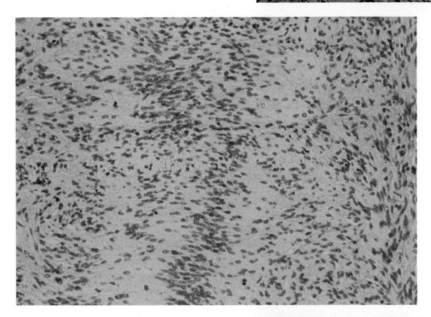

**Figure 31–4.** This photomicrograph of a femoral tumor from a 16-year-old female shows the classic palisading of the nuclei of the spindle cells evident in neurilemmomas of peripheral nerves.

**Figure 31–5.** At high magnification cytologic atypia may be seen in neurilemmomas, as is evident in this mandibular lesion. Mitotic activity should essentially be absent in neurilemmomas; this feature helps to distinguish such lesions with "degenerative atypia" from sarcomas.

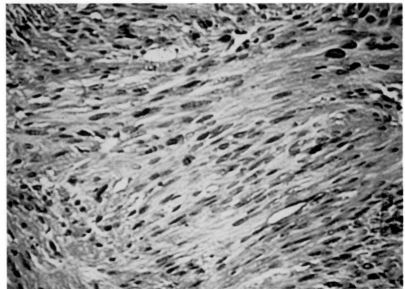

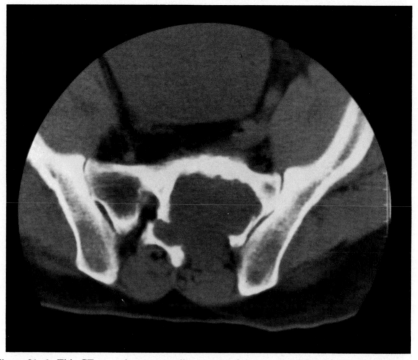

**Figure 31–6.** This CT scan shows a neurilemmoma of the sacrum. The slowly enlarging tumor has eroded and destroyed bone around the left sacral foramen.

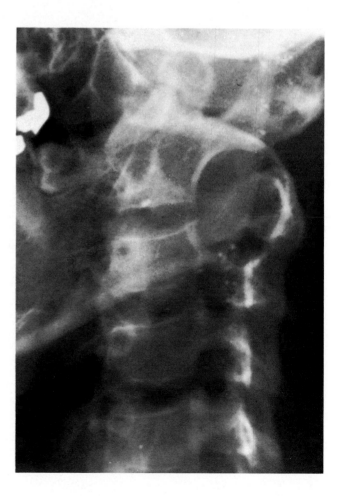

**Figure 31–7.** This neurilemmoma of the cervical nerve root has resulted in marked erosion and expansion of the C2–C3 intervertebral foramen.

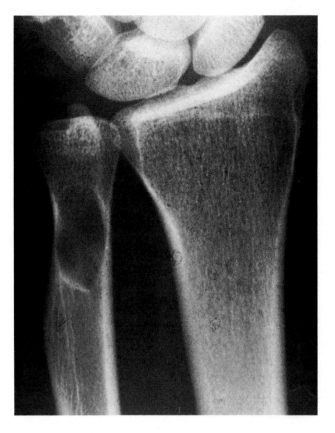

**Figure 31–8.** An intraosseous neurilemmoma of the distal ulna is shown in this radiograph. Very sharp margination is evident, as is the sclerotic rim; these are indications of a benign process.

# CHAPTER 32

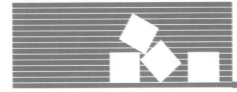

# Adamantinoma

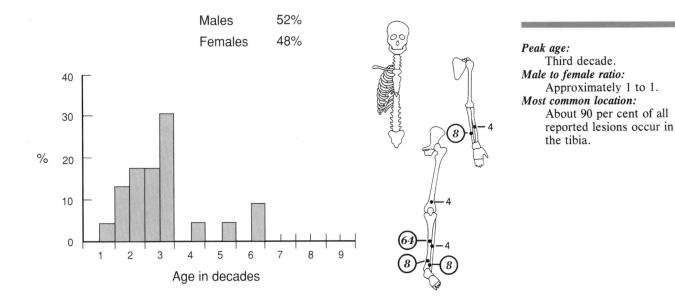

Males 52%
Females 48%

% — Age in decades

*Peak age:*
Third decade.
*Male to female ratio:*
Approximately 1 to 1.
*Most common location:*
About 90 per cent of all reported lesions occur in the tibia.

■ **Clinical Symptoms**

1. Pain is the most common initial symptom.
2. A mass lesion is rarely the initial symptom.
3. The duration of symptoms may be from several months to many years.

■ **Clinical Signs**

1. A mass lesion is the only usual finding on physical examination.

■ **Major Radiographic Features**

1. The lesion occurs in the diaphysis of the tibia.
2. Eccentric lucencies are connected by sclerosis.
3. A dominant central lesion is present.
4. Expansion of the affected bone is common.
5. Multicentricity of the lesion may be present.
6. The fibula may be affected as well.

■ **Radiographic Differential Diagnosis**

1. Osteofibrous dysplasia.
2. Fibrous dysplasia.
3. Fibroma.

■ **Pathologic Features**

*Gross*

1. These tumors tend to be well circumscribed at their periphery and arranged in a lobulated fashion.
2. The tumor is generally gray or white in color.
3. The consistency varies from firm and fibrous to soft.
4. Cystic spaces containing blood or straw-colored fluid may be encountered.

*Microscopic*

1. The tumors may show a myriad of histologic pat-

terns; however, they share an epithelioid low-power pattern.

2. The most common pattern is that of epithelioid islands of cells with peripheral columnar cells showing nuclear palisading.

3. Toward the center of the epithelioid islands, the cells are arranged in a looser pattern with spindling (stellate reticulum-like appearance).

4. Hypocellular fibrous connective tissue occupies the space between the epithelioid islands, and disorganized bone may be seen in these regions, resulting in a pattern that mimics osteofibrous dysplasia.

5. The epithelioid islands may show squamous cytologic features and even keratin production.

6. A vascular pattern with the spaces merging into the epithelial islands is common.

7. The tumor may be purely spindle-celled, mimicking fibrosarcoma; however, a cortical location and a lack of cytologic atypia should suggest a diagnosis of adamantinoma.

## ■ Pathologic Differential Diagnosis

Benign lesions:
1. Osteofibrous dysplasia.
2. Fibrous dysplasia.

Malignant lesions:
1. Metastatic carcinoma.
2. Hemangioendothelial sarcoma.

## ■ Treatment

**Primary Modality:** en bloc removal with a wide surgical margin. Reconstruction of the bone can be achieved with an intercalary allograft or vascularized fibular graft. Amputation may be necessary for large or recurrent lesions.

**Other Possible Approaches:** Simple excision with a marginal margin is discouraged because of a high recurrence rate. Therapeutic lymph node dissection has occasionally been necessary for metastatic disease.

## References

Campanacci M, Giunti A, Bertoni F, et al: Adamantinoma of the long bones: the experience at the Istituto Ortopedico Rizzoli. Am J Surg Pathol 5:533–542, 1981.

Knapp RH, Wick MR, Scheithauer BW, and Unni KK: Adamantinoma of bone: an electron microscopic and immunohistochemical study. Virchows Arch (Pathol Anat) 398:75–86, 1982.

Rosai J, and Pinkus GS: Immunohistochemical demonstration of epithelial differentiation in adamantinoma of the tibia. Am J Surg Pathol 6:427–434, 1982.

Weiss SW, and Dorfman HD: Adamantinoma of long bones: an analysis of nine new cases with emphasis on metastasizing lesions and fibrous dysplasia-like changes. Hum Pathol 8:141–153, 1977.

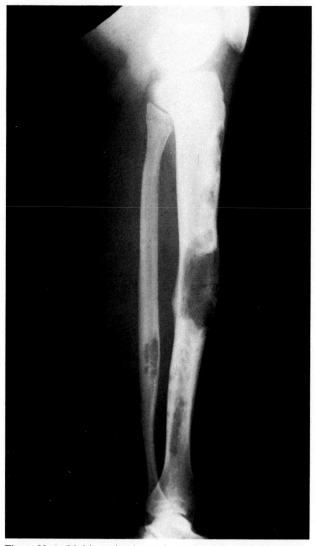

**Figure 32–1.** Multicentric adamantinoma involving the tibia and fibula is shown in this x-ray of the lower extremity. Multiple lytic areas with surrounding sclerosis are present. Note the dominant central expansile lesion.

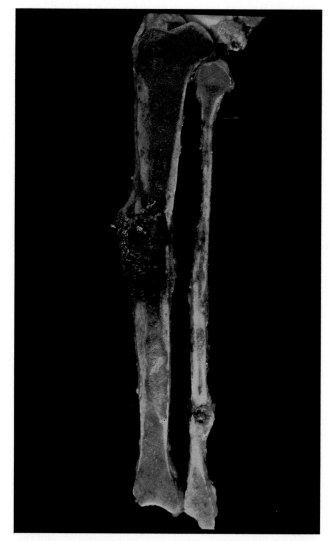

**Figure 32–2.** The bisected gross specimen in this case reveals the involvement of both the tibia and fibula, as was shown in Figure 32–1. Such multicentric disease is not uncommon; indeed, this gross appearance is virtually diagnostic. The multicentric nature of the disease may explain recurrences in cases treated with marginal excision.

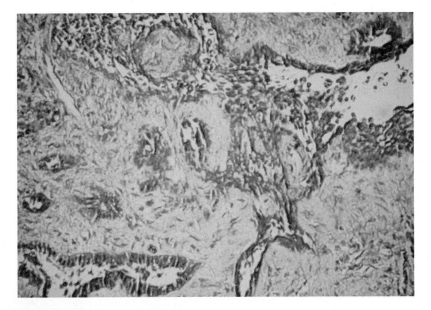

**Figure 32–3.** The low-power pattern of adamantinoma is that of a lesion composed of islands of epithelioid cells lying within a hypocellular fibrous connective tissue. At the periphery of these islands is a palisading of the nuclei. Toward the center of the islands, the cells have a looser arrangement and a more stellate appearance (so-called stellate reticulum).

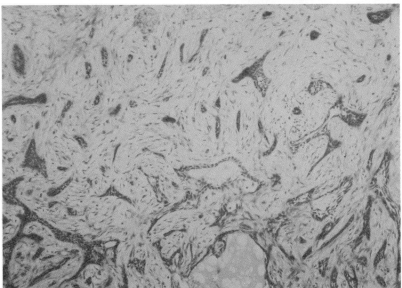

**Figure 32–4.** Some adamantinomas contain more open spaces; when these are blood-filled the appearance may mimic that of a vascular neoplasm.

**Figure 32–5.** Squamous differentiation, as is shown in this case, may be so prominent as to mimic the appearance of a squamous cell carcinoma. Other tumors may appear glandular and therefore present the appearance of metastatic adenocarcinoma.

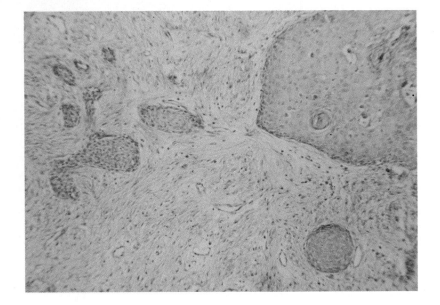

**Figure 32–7.** Multiple small cortical lucencies are apparent in this example of an adamantinoma involving the tibia. The lucencies are connected by sclerotic regions.

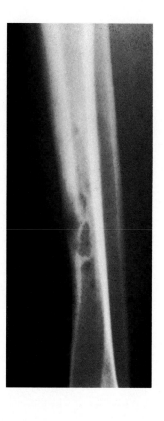

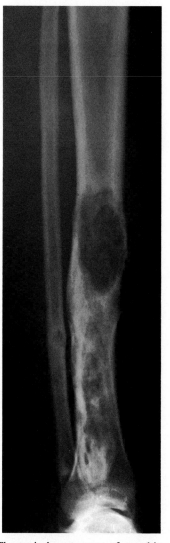

**Figure 32–6.** The typical appearance of a multicentric adamantinoma involving the tibia and fibula is shown in this x-ray. The dominant lesion involves the diaphysis of the tibia and is centrally located.

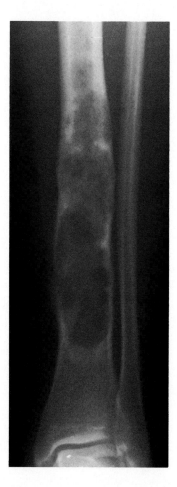

**Figure 32–8.** Adamantinomas are slow-growing lesions and as such may result in significant expansion of the affected bone prior to diagnosis of the lesion. This example shows diaphyseal expansion of the tibia with a sclerotic margin, another feature indicating slow growth.

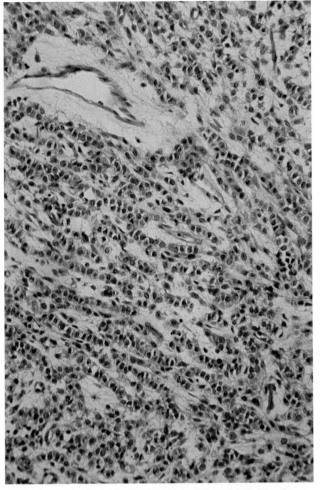

**Figure 32–9.** At times the arrangement of the epithelioid cells may give rise to a single-file pattern, mimicking poorly differentiated adenocarcinoma. This tumor had been present in the tibia for 50 years.

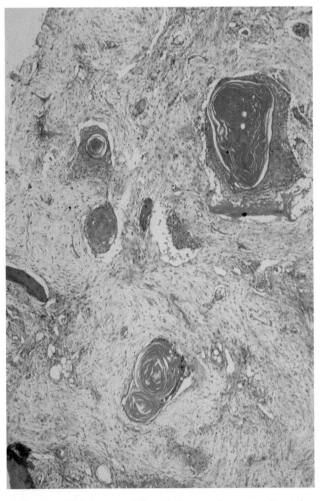

**Figure 32–10.** Squamous differentiation may be so prominent that squamous pearl formation occurs. Such cases may show a deceptively bland cytologic appearance and suggest the diagnosis of squamous cell carcinoma arising in chronic osteomyelitis.

# CHAPTER 33

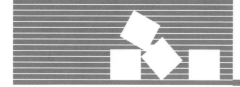

# Giant Cell Tumor

Males      44%
Females     56%

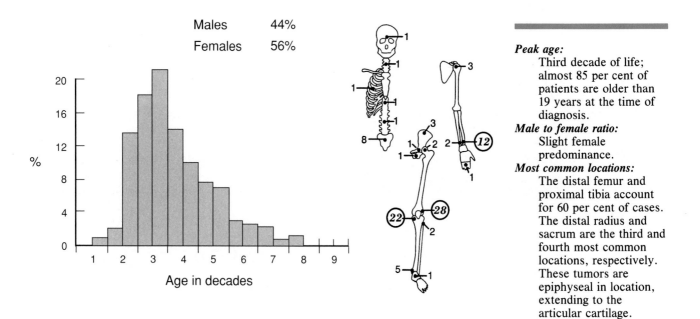

**Peak age:**
Third decade of life; almost 85 per cent of patients are older than 19 years at the time of diagnosis.

**Male to female ratio:**
Slight female predominance.

**Most common locations:**
The distal femur and proximal tibia account for 60 per cent of cases. The distal radius and sacrum are the third and fourth most common locations, respectively. These tumors are epiphyseal in location, extending to the articular cartilage.

## ■ Clinical Symptoms

1. Pain of variable severity is almost uniformly present.
2. Approximately 75 per cent of patients discover a swelling in the region of the affected bone.
3. Pathologic fracture may occur.
4. Limitation of range of motion of the joint adjacent to the affected bone may be noticed.
5. Weakness of the extremity containing the affected bone may be present.

## ■ Clinical Signs

1. Eighty per cent of patients present with a tender, palpable mass.
2. Regional musculature may show atrophic changes secondary to disuse.

## ■ Major Radiographic Features

1. The lesion is purely lytic and epiphyseal in location, extending to the end of the bone.
2. There is neither sclerosis at the periphery of the lesion nor periosteal reaction.
3. Although the tumor is classically epiphyseal in location, it may also arise in an apophysis.
4. The radiographic appearance may mimic that of a malignant tumor.

## ■ Radiographic Differential Diagnosis

1. Chondroblastoma.
2. Osteosarcoma.
3. Fibrosarcoma.
4. Malignant fibrous histiocytoma.

## ■ Pathologic Features

### Gross

1. The curetted fragments of tissue are soft and friable.
2. The color of the lesion varies from gray-brown to reddish; there may also be yellow regions containing numerous lipid-laden macrophages.
3. Necrosis with resultant cyst formation may be seen.
4. Tumors may be confined to the bone or may have extended through the cortex into the surrounding soft tissues.

### Microscopic

1. Although these tumors may show regions of necrosis and cyst formation, in general they have a uniform pattern of growth on low magnification.
2. Multinucleated giant cells lie scattered uniformly in a "sea" of mononuclear cells, which are round to oval in shape.
3. On higher magnification, the nuclei of the mononuclear cells and those of the multinucleated giant cells are similar in appearance and uniform in their cytologic characteristics.
4. Mitotic figures may be quite abundant.
5. The tumor lacks matrix production; when pathologic fracture has occurred, however, the reactive new bone formation may alter the histology of the tumor.

## ■ Pathologic Differential Diagnosis

Benign lesions:
1. Giant cell reparative granuloma (giant cell reaction).
2. Aneurysmal bone cyst.
3. Chondroblastoma.
Malignant lesions:
1. Malignant fibrous histiocytoma.
2. Malignancy in giant cell tumor (malignant giant cell tumor).
3. Osteosarcoma containing numerous giant cells.

## ■ Treatment

**Primary Modality:** surgical excision, with the extent of surgery depending on the size and local extent of the tumor. The three primary therapeutic options are (1) curettage and bone grafting for less extensive lesions; (2) resection with bone and joint reconstruction for the very aggressive lesions with associated soft tissue extension, loss of articular cartilage, or pathologic fracture; and (3) curettage and cementation for lesions between these two ends of the spectrum.

**Other Possible Approaches:** cryosurgery or chemical cautery as an adjuvant to curettage and grafting. Radiation therapy should be reserved for surgically inaccessible lesions (e.g., extensive sacral involvement) because of the subsequent risk of malignant "transformation."

### References

Cooper KL, Beabout JW, and Dahlin DC: Giant-cell tumor: ossification in soft tissue implants. Radiology 153:597–602, 1984.

Larsson SE, Lorentzon R, and Boquist L: Giant-cell tumor of bone: a demographic, clinical and histopathological study of all cases recorded in the Swedish Cancer Registry for years 1958 through 1968. J Bone Joint Surg 57A:167–173, 1975.

Marcove RC, Weis LD, Vaghaiwalla MR, et al: Cryosurgery in the treatment of giant cell tumors of bone: a report of 52 consecutive cases. Cancer 41:957–969, 1978.

Peimer CA, Schiller AL, Mankin JH, and Smith RJ: Multicentric giant-cell tumor of bone. J Bone Joint Surg 62A:652–656, 1980.

Picci P, Manfrini M, Zucchi V, et al: Giant-cell tumor of bone in skeletally immature patients. J Bone Joint Surg 65A:486–490, 1983.

Rock MG, Pritchard DJ, and Unni KK: Metastases from histologically benign giant-cell tumor of bone. J Bone Joint Surg 66A:269–274, 1984.

Sanerkin NG: Malignancy, aggressiveness, and recurrence in giant cell tumor of bone. Cancer 46:1641–1649, 1980.

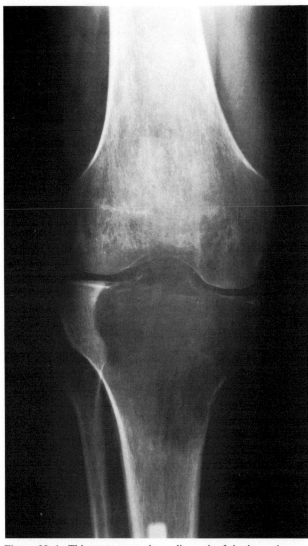

**Figure 33–1.** This anteroposterior radiograph of the knee shows a large, purely lytic, eccentric lesion involving the proximal tibia. The lesion extends to the end of the bone, and there is expansion of the bone and associated cortical destruction. The features are typical of giant cell tumor.

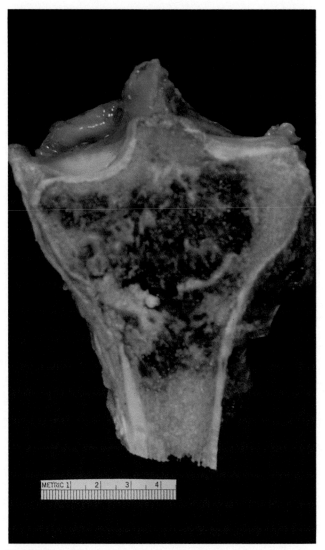

**Figure 33–2.** The gross pathologic appearance of the lesion correlates well with its radiographic appearance in Figure 33–1. The tumor varies in color from brown to yellow and extends to the articular surface.

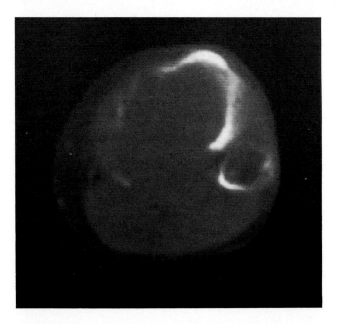

**Figure 33–3.** The CT scan in this case also shows the lesion to be purely lytic, a feature that helps to support a diagnosis of giant cell tumor. Cortical destruction and soft tissue extension, evidence of aggressive behavior, are commonly seen in giant cell tumor.

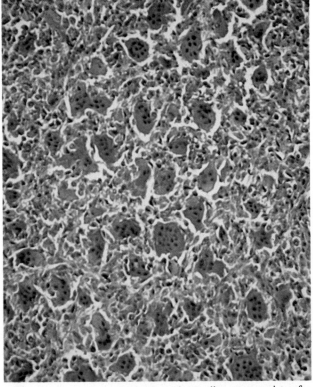

**Figure 33–4.** At low magnification, giant cell tumor consists of a "sea" of mononuclear cells within which multinucleated giant cells are scattered in a uniform manner.

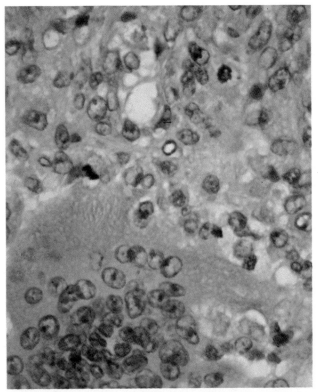

**Figure 33–6.** At high magnification the nuclei of the mononuclear stromal cells are similar to those of the multinucleated giant cells. This feature is evident in this tumor from the proximal humerus. Mitotic activity may be brisk in giant cell tumors.

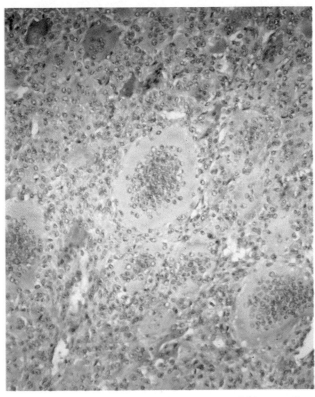

**Figure 33–5.** Although the histologic appearance of this tumor from the proximal humerus is typical of giant cell tumor, the aggressive radiographic features exhibited by the lesion suggested the possibility of telangiectatic osteosarcoma.

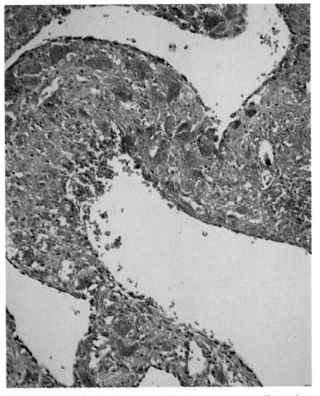

**Figure 33–7.** Secondary aneurysmal bone cyst may complicate giant cell tumor. In cases such as this, the identification of the underlying giant cell tumor may be difficult.

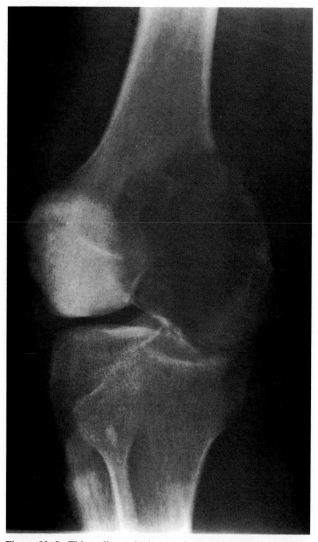

**Figure 33–8.** This radiograph shows a large, eccentric, aggressive-appearing giant cell tumor of the distal femur. The purely lytic nature of the lesion, its extension to the articular surface, and its eccentric location favor a diagnosis of giant cell tumor.

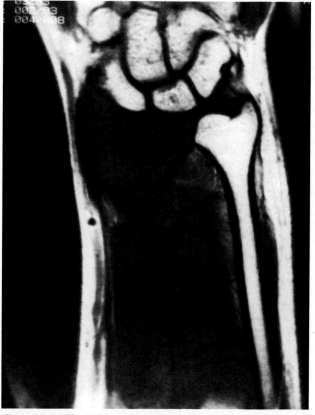

**Figure 33–9.** This MR image of a giant cell tumor of the distal radius demonstrates the utility of this imaging modality, particularly for tumors in peripheral locations. The distal radius is a common site for giant cell tumor.

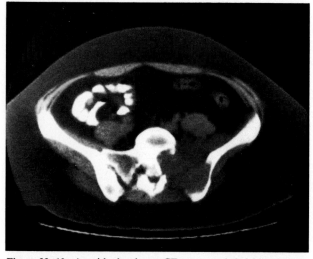

**Figure 33–10.** As with chordoma, CT scans are helpful in detecting giant cell tumors of the sacrum. These tumors (such as the one shown in this radiograph) may cause extensive destruction of the bone, and the soft tissue involvement generally is better appreciated with CT.

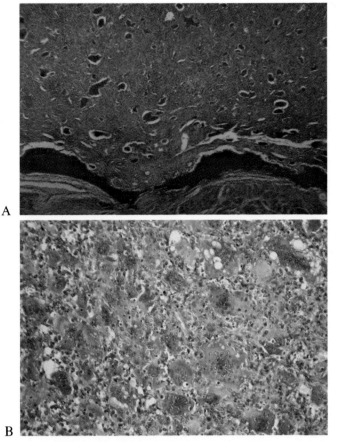

A

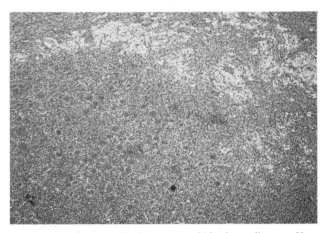

B

**Figure 33–11.** A rim of reactive bone (*A*) frequently surrounds soft tissue recurrences of giant cell tumor. The recurrences—whether osseous, soft tissue, or pulmonary metastases—show the same histologic features as the primary tumor (*B*).

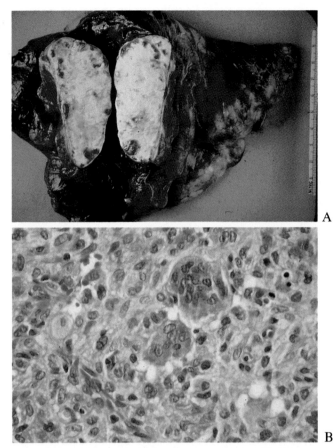

A

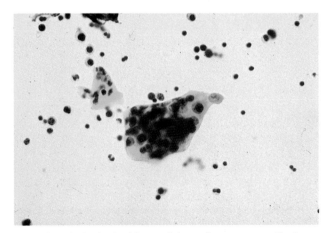

B

**Figure 33–13.** The pulmonary metastases (gross pathologic features, *A*) that rarely complicate the clinical course of treated giant cell tumor exhibit the same cytologic similarity between mononuclear and multinucleated cells as is shown in this photomicrograph (*B*).

**Figure 33–12.** Degeneration is common within giant cell tumor. Xanthomatous change is illustrated in this photomicrograph of a distal femoral tumor.

**Figure 33–14.** Aspiration biopsy of giant cell tumors generally shows numerous multinucleated giant cells, as are seen in this aspirate of a sacral lesion.

# CHAPTER 34

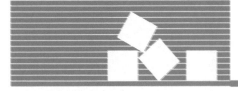

# Chordoma

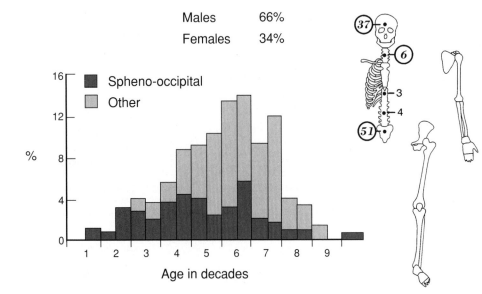

| Males | 66% |
| Females | 34% |

Spheno-occipital
Other

% / Age in decades

**Peak age:**
 Sixth decade.
**Male to female ratio:**
 Approximately 2 to 1.
**Most common locations:**
 The sacrum
 (approximately 50 per
 cent of cases) and the
 spheno-occipital region
 (approximately 35 per
 cent of cases).

## ■ Clinical Symptoms

1. Symptoms and duration are variable and depend on tumor location (sacrum, spheno-occipital, or vertebral); however, they are usually of long duration.
2. Sacral tumors nearly always are associated with pain in the sacral or coccygeal region. Constipation may be experienced.
3. Spheno-occipital tumors generally cause symptoms related to involvement of cranial nerves. Of these, the sixth, seventh, and eighth are the most frequently involved.
4. Vertebral chordomas may cause symptoms owing to nerve root or spinal cord compression.

## ■ Clinical Signs

1. Sacral tumors generally extend anteriorly and thus produce a presacral mass appreciable on rectal examination.

2. Spheno-occipital tumors cause sixth nerve palsy but may also result in seventh and eighth nerve abnormalities. Downward growth may produce a nasopharyngeal mass lesion.
3. Vertebral chordomas give rise to nerve root compression or spinal cord compression signs, but those in the cervical region may also result in symptoms suggestive of a chronic retropharyngeal abscess.

## ■ Major Radiographic Features

1. The lesion is in the sacrum or clivus.
2. Midline destruction is seen. (Regardless of location—sacral, clival, or vertebral—all chordomas are midline lesions.)
3. Poor margination and an associated soft tissue mass are commonly present.
4. Fifty per cent of all chordomas are calcified radiographically.

5. Computed tomography (CT) and magnetic resonance imaging (MRI) are the best modalities to delineate the extent of the lesion.

## ■ Radiographic Differential Diagnosis

1. Metastatic carcinoma.
2. Myeloma.
3. Giant cell tumor.
4. Neurogenic tumor.

## ■ Pathologic Features

### Gross

1. Chordomas generally are soft, grayish tumors that have a gelatinous consistency grossly.
2. The tumor tends to be well circumscribed and may even show gross lobulation.
3. In both the sacral and spheno-occipital regions, the tumor tends to elevate the periosteum of the affected bone, extending into the presacral and cranial cavities, respectively.

### Microscopic

1. On low magnification chordomas characteristically are arranged in a lobulated fashion, with fibrous septa separating the lobules.
2. The tumor generally is arranged in chords or strands of cells.
3. Between the chords of cells is abundant intercellular mucoid matrix.
4. On higher magnification the cells have abundant eosinophilic vacuolated cytoplasm (physaliferous cells). The boundaries between cells in the strands are indistinct, resulting in a syncytial quality.
5. In the spheno-occipital region, some tumors show a histology very similar to that of chondrosarcoma (chondroid chondroma).

## ■ Pathologic Differential Diagnosis

Benign lesions:
1. Chondromyxoid fibroma.
Malignant lesions:
1. Metastatic carcinoma.
2. Chondrosarcoma.

## ■ Treatment

**Primary Modality:** en bloc resection with a marginal or wide margin; sacrificing involved nerve roots provides the best chance for cure. Sacral lesions below the third sacral vertebra can be removed with a posterior approach; lesions above this level are approached both anteriorly and posteriorly.

**Other Possible Approaches:** Adjuvant radiation is utilized for narrow or contaminated margins and surgically inaccessible lesions. Radiation therapy is particularly helpful for tumors in the spheno-occipital region.

## References

Chambers PW, and Schwinn CP: Chordoma: a clinicopathologic study of metastasis. Am J Clin Pathol 72:765–776, 1979.

Eriksson B, Gunterberg B, and Kindblom LG: Chordoma: a clinicopathologic and prognostic study of a Swedish national series. Acta Orthop Scand 52:49–58, 1981.

Kaiser TE, Pritchard DJ, and Unni KK: Clinicopathologic study of sacrococcygeal chordoma. Cancer 53:2574–2578, 1984.

Mindell ER: Current concepts review: chordoma. J Bone Joint Surg 63A:501–505, 1981.

Volpe R, and Mazabraud A: A clinicopathologic review of 25 cases of chordoma (a pleomorphic and metastasizing neoplasm). Am J Surg Pathol 7:161–170, 1983.

Wold LE, and Laws ER Jr: Cranial chordomas in children and young adults. J Neurosurg 59:1043–1047, 1983.

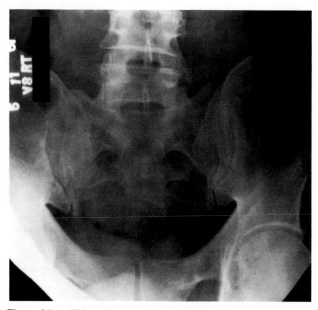

**Figure 34–1.** This radiograph illustrates how difficult it may be to demonstrate a chordoma in the sacrum with a routine anteroposterior view.

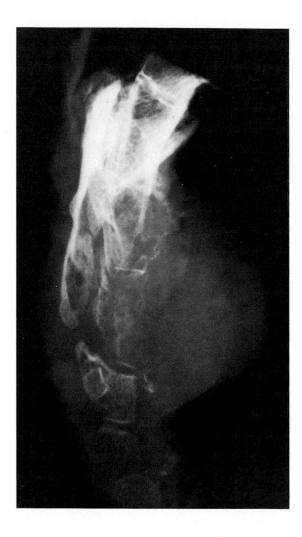

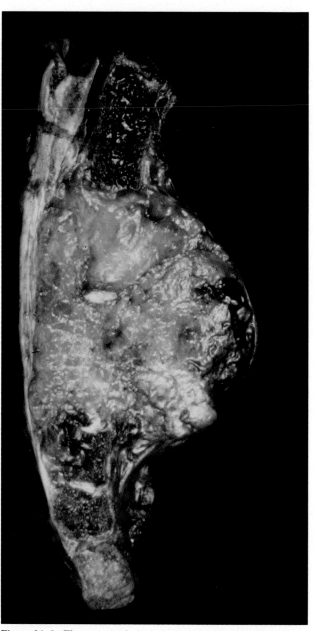

**Figure 34–2.** The gross pathologic features in this case (also shown in Fig. 34–1) demonstrate destruction of a significant portion of the sacrum and extension of the tumor into the presacral space.

**Figure 34–3.** The specimen radiogram exhibits the same features as seen in the gross specimen. Lateral radiographs of the pelvis may help to visualize a sacral chordoma, as do CT and MRI analysis.

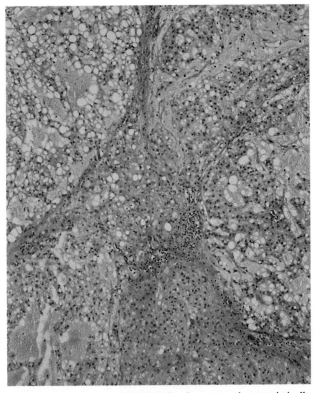

**Figure 34–4.** At low magnification chordomas are characteristically lobulated tumors, as this photomicrograph shows.

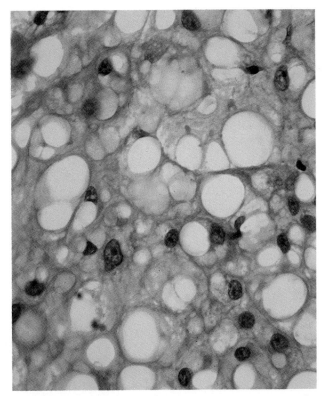

**Figure 34–6.** At high magnification the cytologic features show that the cells have abundant vacuolated cytoplasm. Such cells have been termed "physaliferous."

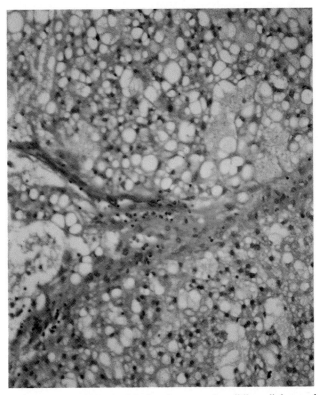

**Figure 34–5.** Within the lobules the tumor is mildly cellular, and numerous cytoplasmic vacuoles are identifiable even at medium magnification. Chording of the cells is a feature that varies from tumor to tumor and need not be prominent.

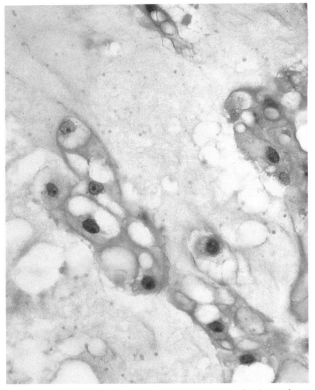

**Figure 34–7.** Chording of the cells, as shown in this photomicrograph, is a feature that can result in a histologic pattern similar to a mucinous adenocarcinoma.

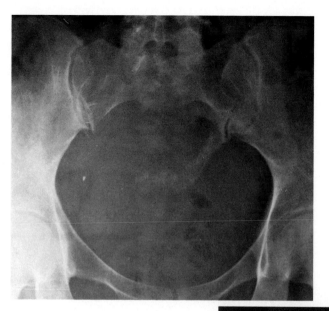

**Figure 34–8.** This radiograph shows a chordoma presenting as a large, poorly marginated, midline, destructive tumor of the sacrum. An area of central calcification is present.

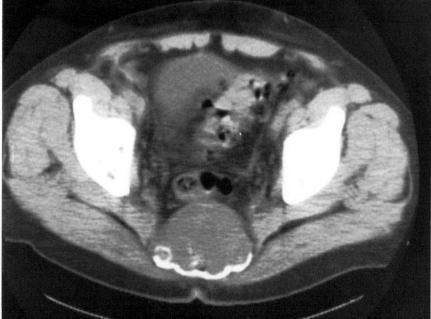

**Figure 34–9.** This CT scan shows the typical features of a sacral chordoma, with bony destruction and anterior extension of the lesion.

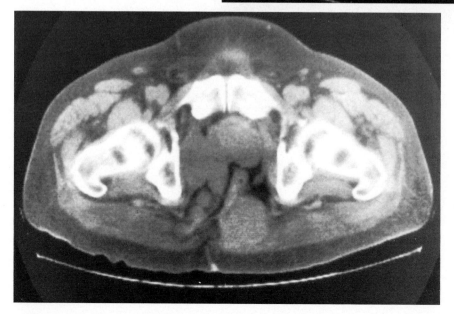

**Figure 34–10.** Multiple soft tissue nodules of recurrent chordoma are identifiable in this CT scan. These tumors have a propensity for such recurrences, and CT or MRI usually is needed to detect them.

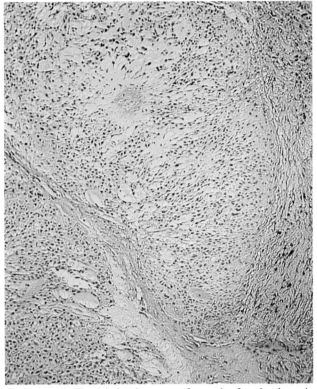

**Figure 34–11.** The lobulated pattern of growth of a chordoma is evident in this sacral tumor. Soft tissue extensions of the tumor maintain this pattern.

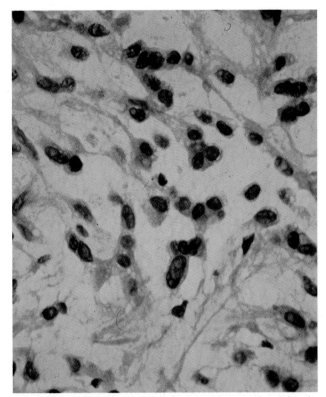

**Figure 34–13.** Chording is also evident in this tumor involving the seventh thoracic vertebra. Although some mesenchymal and even epithelial tumors may exhibit a similar pattern of chorded growth, the diagnosis of chordoma is only valid for midline tumors.

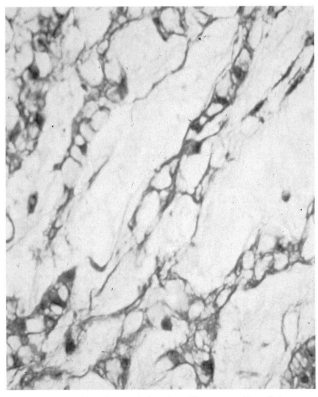

**Figure 34–12.** Chording and the physaliferous quality of the cytoplasm are evident in this photomicrograph.

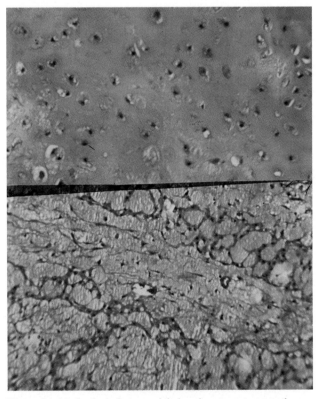

**Figure 34–14.** In the spheno-occipital region some tumors show a mixture of chondroid and chordoid features histologically. Such tumors have been termed "chondroid chordomas."

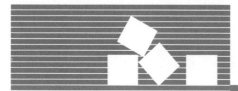

# CHAPTER 35

# Ewing's Sarcoma

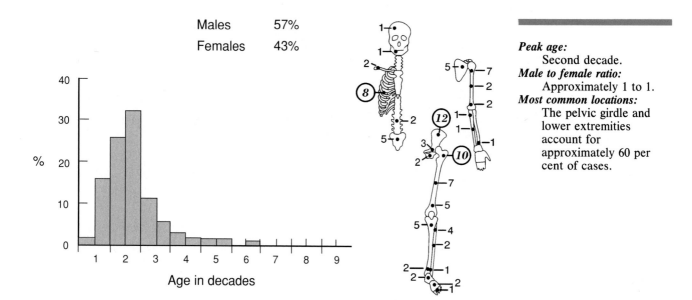

Males 57%
Females 43%

%

40

30

20

10

0

1 2 3 4 5 6 7 8 9

Age in decades

*Peak age:*
Second decade.
*Male to female ratio:*
Approximately 1 to 1.
*Most common locations:*
The pelvic girdle and lower extremities account for approximately 60 per cent of cases.

## ■ Clinical Symptoms

1. Local pain is the first symptom in 50 per cent of patients. Although it may be intermittent at first, pain tends to increase in severity over time.
2. Swelling is commonly present at the time of diagnosis but is rarely the first symptom.
3. Fever and other constitutional symptoms suggestive of an infection may be present.

## ■ Clinical Signs

1. A palpable, tender mass lesion is found.
2. Fever and an increased erythrocyte sedimentation rate may be seen.
3. Anemia and leukocytosis may also be present.

## ■ Major Radiographic Features

1. The tumor most commonly presents as an extensive diaphyseal lesion.

2. The lesion has a permeative pattern of growth and is poorly marginated.
3. The lesion may be lytic or sclerotic or it may have regions of both lysis and sclerosis evident radiographically.
4. Characteristically, there is prominent periosteal new bone formation.
5. A soft tissue mass most commonly accompanies the osseous lesion.
6. An isotope bone scan, computed tomography (CT), and magnetic resonance imaging (MRI) are helpful in defining the lesion.

## ■ Radiographic Differential Diagnosis

1. Malignant lymphoma.
2. Osteosarcoma.
3. Osteomyelitis.
4. Histiocytosis X (Langerhans' cell granulomatosis).

## ■ Pathologic Features

### Gross

1. The tumor is characteristically grayish-white in color.
2. The tumor is moist and glistening.
3. The tumor may be almost liquid in consistency and can mimic the appearance of pus.

### Microscopic

1. The low-power appearance is that of a ''small round cell tumor'' with little intercellular stroma.
2. Between the areas of highly cellular tumor, fibrous strands may be identified that compartmentalize the tumor.
3. At high magnification the cells are uniform and round to oval in shape.
4. The nuclei are round to oval and have a delicate, finely dispersed chromatin pattern.
5. Nucleoli, if present, are inconspicuous.
6. Mitotic figures are not abundant.
7. The majority of tumors have glycogen identifiable in the cytoplasm (periodic acid-Schiff–positive and diastase-sensitive).
8. The tumor is reticulin-poor and does not show evidence of matrix production.

## ■ Pathologic Differential Diagnosis

Benign lesions:
1. Chronic osteomyelitis.

Malignant lesions:
1. Malignant lymphoma.
2. Mesenchymal chondrosarcoma.
3. Small cell osteosarcoma.
4. Metastatic neuroblastoma.

## ■ Treatment

**Primary Modality:** radiation therapy to control the primary lesion, with 5000 to 6000 rads delivered to the whole bone. An effort is made to avoid irradiating an actively growing physis. Combination chemotherapy to control occult systemic disease is used in combination with the radiotherapy.

**Other Possible Approaches:** preoperative chemotherapy followed by resection with or without postoperative radiation therapy. Increased emphasis is being given to the addition of surgical treatment to the overall therapy of Ewing's tumor.

### References

Bacci G, Picci P, Gitelis S, et al: The treatment of localized Ewing's sarcoma: the experience at the Istituto Ortopedico Rizzoli in 163 cases treated with and without adjuvant chemotherapy. Cancer 49:1561–1570, 1982.

Kissane JM, Askin FB, Fokulkes M, et al: Ewing's sarcoma of bone: clinicopathologic aspects of 303 cases from the Intergroup Ewing's Sarcoma Study. Hum Pathol 14:773–779, 1983.

Mendenhall CM, Marcus RB Jr, Enneking WF, et al: The prognostic significance of soft tissue extension in Ewing's sarcoma. Cancer 51:913–917, 1983.

Nascimento AG, Unni KK, Pritchard DJ, et al: A clinicopathologic study of 20 cases of large-cell (atypical) Ewing's sarcoma of bone. Am J Surg Pathol 4:29–36, 1980.

Rosen G, Caparros B, Nirenberg A, et al: Ewing's sarcoma: ten-year experience with adjuvant chemotherapy. Cancer 47:2204–2213, 1981.

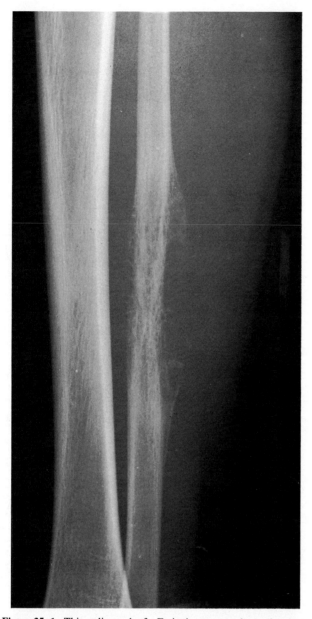

**Figure 35–1.** This radiograph of a Ewing's sarcoma shows the characteristic lytic appearance of such tumors. A diaphyseal location, as in this case involving the fibula, is most common. The periosteum is generally elevated in such cases, resulting in Codman's triangle and an associated soft tissue mass.

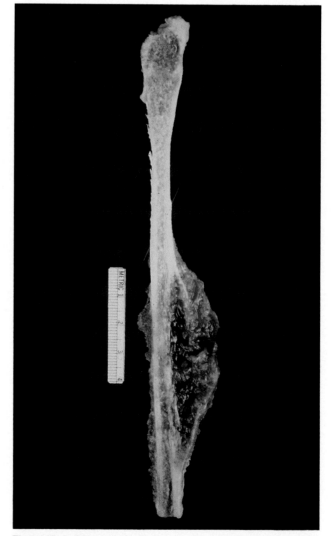

**Figure 35–2.** The gross pathologic features of this fibular Ewing's sarcoma correlate well with the radiographic features shown in Figure 35–1. The lesional tissue is frequently soft and hemorrhagic, as in this case. A small incisional biopsy may yield a loose gray-white tissue that mimics the gross features of an osteomyelitis.

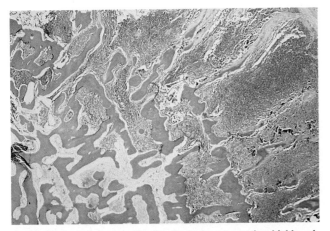

**Figure 35–3.** At low magnification Ewing's sarcoma is a highly cellular tumor composed of small round cells. The periosteum is elevated by this cellular proliferation, resulting in a layering of periosteal new bone that may appear as an "onion skin" radiographically. The reactive new bone is shown in this photomicrograph.

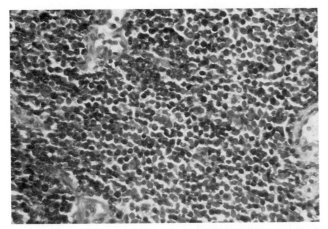

**Figure 35–4.** At higher magnification Ewing's sarcoma is composed of small round cells; frequently, however, two cell types are identifiable. The nuclei of the most prominent type are round with a regular chromatin pattern; if nucleoli are present they are indistinct. The second cell type contains a dark, hyperchromatic nucleus and is thought to represent a degenerative change.

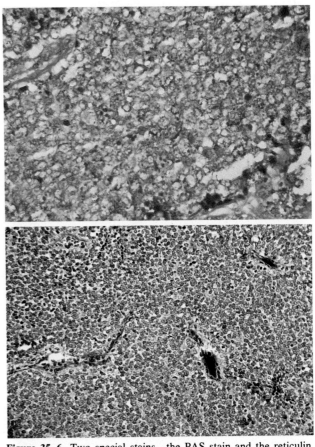

A

B

**Figure 35–6.** Two special stains—the PAS stain and the reticulin stain—are helpful in confirming the diagnosis of Ewing's sarcoma. Ewing's sarcoma is generally, but not uniformly, PAS-positive (*A*) and reticulin-poor (*B*).

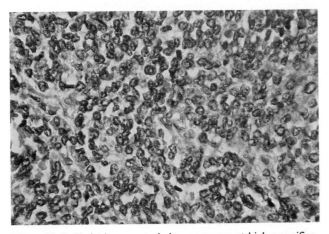

**Figure 35–5.** Ewing's sarcoma is homogeneous at high magnification, and no matrix is identifiable within the tumor. In contrast, small-cell osteosarcoma should have identifiable osteoid within the tumor.

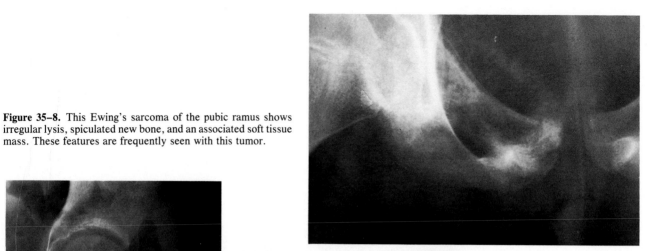

**Figure 35–8.** This Ewing's sarcoma of the pubic ramus shows irregular lysis, spiculated new bone, and an associated soft tissue mass. These features are frequently seen with this tumor.

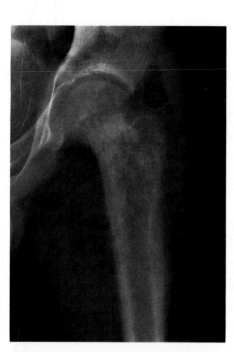

**Figure 35–7.** This radiograph shows a Ewing's sarcoma of the proximal femur. The lesion is long and poorly marginated. The multilamina or "onion skin" periosteal reaction is evident.

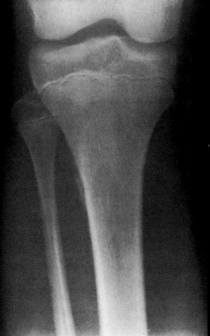

**Figure 35–9.** This plane radiograph shows only new bone formation associated with a Ewing's sarcoma of the proximal tibia.

A

B

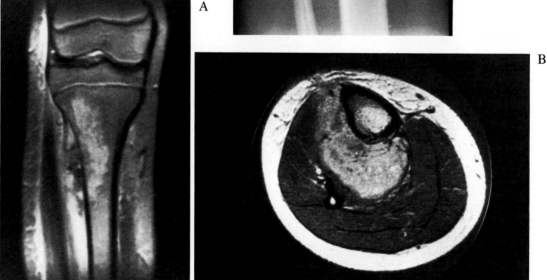

**Figure 35–10.** Although the plane radiographic features are unimpressive (see Fig. 35–9), coronal MRI shows a fairly large intramedullary tumor with cortical destruction and elevation of the periosteum (*A*). Axial MRI of the same tumor shows a large soft tissue mass typical of this tumor (*B*). This case demonstrates the utility of CT and MRI in the evaluation of cases that are inconspicuous on plane radiographic evaluation.

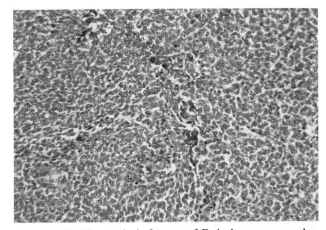

**Figure 35–12.** The cytologic features of Ewing's sarcoma are homogeneous, as this photomicrograph shows. Foci of necrosis may be present.

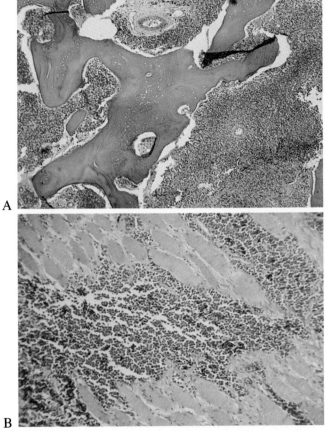

A

B

**Figure 35–11.** These photomicrographs illustrate the permeative nature of the pattern of growth of Ewing's sarcoma, whether it is in bone (*A*) or involves the soft tissues adjacent to the affected bone (*B*).

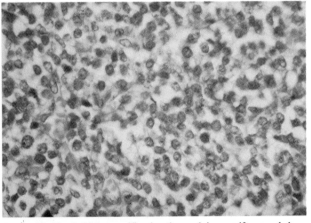

**Figure 35–13.** At high magnification the nuclei are uniform and show a finely granular chromatin pattern.

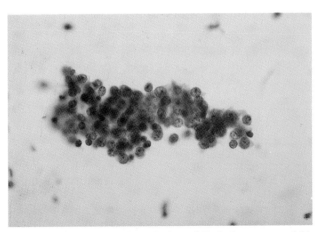

**Figure 35–14.** Fine needle aspiration of Ewing's sarcoma yields small uniform cells, which may be found in clusters but are generally noncohesive in smear preparations. Although diagnosis of the primary tumor with this technique is possible, its main utility is in confirming metastatic disease, as in this case of a transthoracic needle aspirate in a patient with a primary tumor in the ilium.

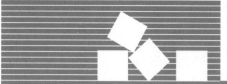

# CHAPTER 36

# Malignancy in Giant Cell Tumor
# (Malignant Giant Cell Tumor)

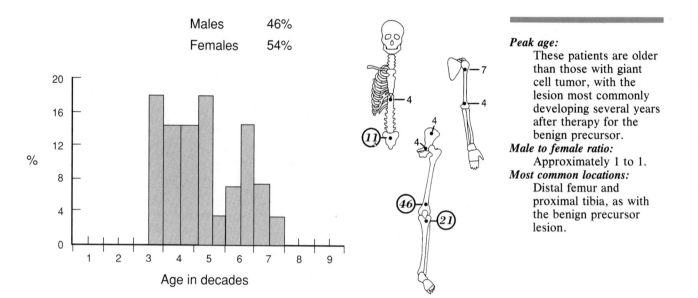

Males    46%

Females   54%

Age in decades

*Peak age:*
These patients are older than those with giant cell tumor, with the lesion most commonly developing several years after therapy for the benign precursor.

*Male to female ratio:*
Approximately 1 to 1.

*Most common locations:*
Distal femur and proximal tibia, as with the benign precursor lesion.

■ **Clinical Symptoms**

1. Pain is the most common symptom.
2. Nearly all patients give a history of a previous giant cell tumor having been treated more than 10 years (on average) prior to their recent onset of pain.
3. Seventy-five per cent of patients have received prior radiation therapy as part of their treatment for the giant cell tumor.
4. Only rarely is an abrupt change in the symptoms related to the development of a "malignant giant cell tumor" in a patient who has *not* received prior radiation therapy.

■ **Clinical Signs**

1. A tender mass lesion in the region of a previously treated giant cell tumor is commonly present on physical examination.
2. Cutaneous changes from prior radiation therapy are commonly found.

■ **Major Radiographic Features**

1. A de novo malignant giant cell tumor has the same radiographic appearance as a benign giant cell tumor, and the two cannot be distinguished.
2. A secondary malignant giant cell tumor is usu-

ally seen many years (average of 13 years) after treatment that included radiation therapy.

3. Serial changes that occur more than three years after the original treatment are highly suspect for secondary malignant giant cell tumor.

■ **Radiographic Differential Diagnosis**

1. Benign giant cell tumor.
2. Recurrent giant cell tumor.
3. Osteomyelitis.

■ **Pathologic Features**

*Gross*

1. The tumor expands the end of the bone and generally has broken through the cortex.
2. Zones of necrosis are identifiable; however, necrosis can be seen in benign giant cell tumors as well.
3. Extension into the surrounding soft tissue is generally present.
4. Hemorrhagic foci may also be identified.

*Microscopic*

1. At low magnification the tumor is hypercellular and generally is composed of spindle cells.
2. Matrix production may be but generally is not present.
3. The arrangement of the spindle cells may be in a "herring bone," storiform, or haphazard pattern.
4. At higher magnification the spindle cells show marked pleomorphism and nuclear atypia characterized by variation in their size, shape, and staining qualities.

5. In general, mitotic activity is brisk.
6. Most commonly, no residual benign giant cell tumor is identifiable in the lesion. On rare occasions, however, zones of otherwise typical giant cell tumor may be identified adjacent to the high-grade sarcoma.

■ **Pathologic Differential Diagnosis**

Benign lesions:
1. Giant cell tumor.
2. Metaphyseal fibrous defect (fibroma).
Malignant lesions:
1. Osteosarcoma.
2. Fibrosarcoma.
3. Malignant fibrous histiocytoma.

■ **Treatment**

**Primary Modality:** preoperative chemotherapy and wide surgical resection. Aggressive behavior and extensive involvement often mandate amputation to achieve an adequate margin.

**Other Possible Approaches:** chemotherapy, radiation therapy for surgically inaccessible lesions, and thoracotomy for metastatic pulmonary disease.

### References

Hutter RVP, Worcester JN Jr, Francis KC, et al: Benign and malignant giant cell tumors of bone: a clinicopathological analysis of the natural history of the disease. Cancer *15*:653–690, 1962.

Nascimento AG, Huvos AG, and Marcove RC: Primary malignant giant cell tumor of bone: a study of eight cases and review of the literature. Cancer *44*:1393–1402, 1979.

Sanerkin NG: Malignancy, aggressiveness, and recurrence in giant cell tumor of bone. Cancer *46*:1641–1649, 1980.

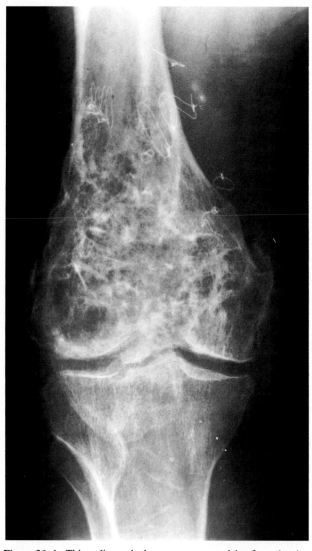

**Figure 36–1.** This radiograph shows a sarcoma arising from the site of a prior benign giant cell tumor. The development of the sarcoma is often obscured by the distortion caused by the previous tumor. Serial studies are essential to confidently make the diagnosis in many cases.

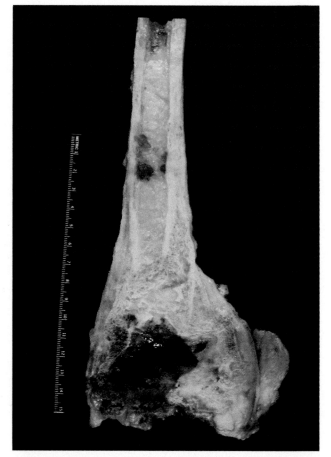

**Figure 36–2.** The gross specimen of the tumor seen in Figure 36–1 is shown. The distal femur has been replaced by a firm fibrous tumor, which has destroyed the medial cortex of the femur. This sarcoma, which showed the histologic pattern of growth of a fibrosarcoma, occurred in a patient who had received radiation therapy for a giant cell tumor 12 years previously.

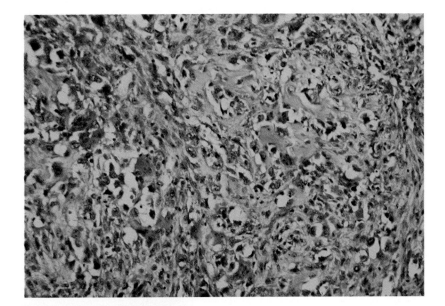

**Figure 36–3.** In contrast with benign giant cell tumors, in which the mononuclear cells contain nuclei similar to those in the multinucleated giant cells, malignancies arising in giant cell tumors show marked nuclear pleomorphism, as this photomicrograph illustrates.

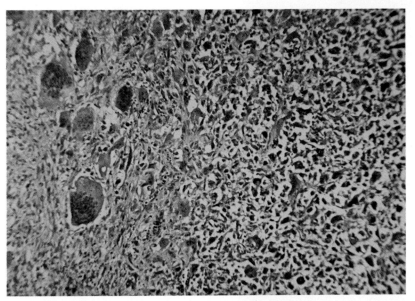

**Figure 36–4.** Although malignancy is rarely identified de novo in giant cell tumors, when such cases are encountered both a benign giant cell tumor component and a sarcoma should be histologically identifiable. This photomicrograph shows a distal femoral tumor from a 28-year-old male that radiographically was classic for a benign giant cell tumor. Histologically the lesion shows a pattern typical of benign giant cell tumor, as well as a sarcomatous component.

**Figure 36–5.** Malignancies that arise in the region of a prior giant cell tumor almost uniformly consist of spindle-shaped cells. This tumor shows some features of a malignant fibrous histiocytoma. Osseous and chondroid matrix production may also be evident in these tumors.

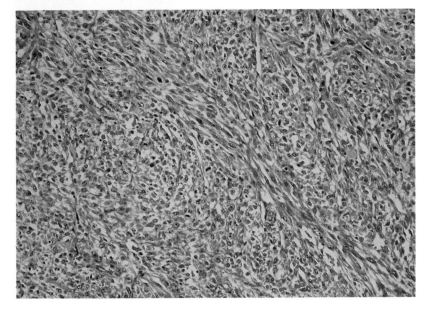

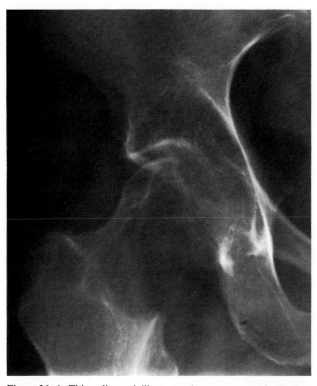

**Figure 36–6.** This radiograph illustrates the appearance of a de novo malignant giant cell tumor of the proximal femur, characterized by an aggressive appearance and lytic destruction extending to the bone end. Benign giant cell tumors may also cause this type of change.

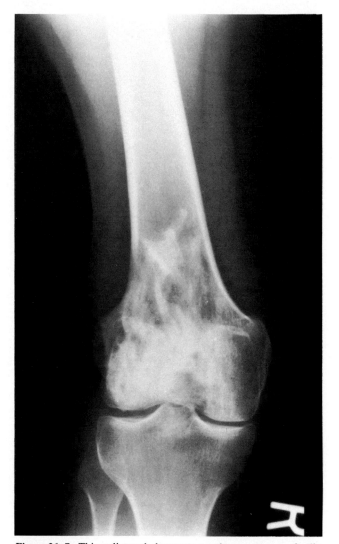

**Figure 36–7.** This radiograph demonstrates the appearance of a distal femur 16 years after curettage, grafting, and radiation for a benign giant cell tumor.

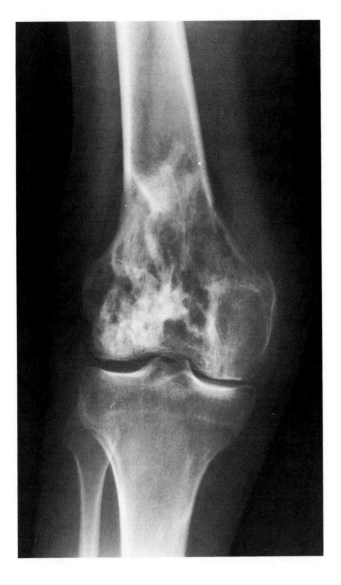

**Figure 36–8.** In this view, taken five months after the radiograph shown in Figure 36–7, the appearance of the lesion has changed. Lytic destruction due to secondary fibrosarcoma has developed.

# CHAPTER 37

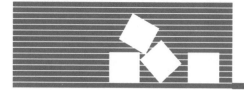

# Paget's Sarcoma

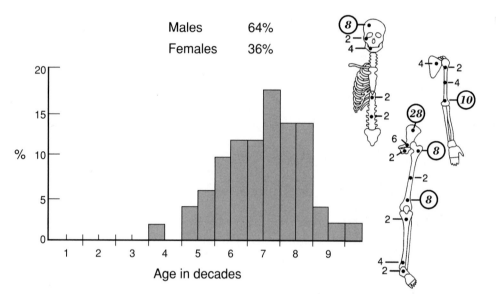

Males 64%
Females 36%

Age in decades

*Peak age:*
  Elderly patients.
*Male to female ratio:*
  Approximately 2 to 1.
*Most common locations:*
  Innominate bone and
  humerus.

## ■ Clinical Symptoms

1. Pain is felt in the affected region. An increase in pain in one bone in a patient with Paget's disease should arouse suspicion of the development of a sarcoma.
2. A swelling may be due to soft tissue extension of the tumor.

## ■ Clinical Signs

1. A painful mass lesion is felt in the region of the affected bone.
2. Symptoms are rapidly progressive.

## ■ Major Radiographic Features

1. Most tumors are purely lytic, although sclerotic and mixed lesions do occur.
2. The bone of origin usually shows changes of Paget's disease.
3. The tumor extends into the surrounding soft tissue.

4. There is a pattern of geographic bone destruction.
5. Computed tomography (CT) or magnetic resonance imaging (MRI) may be useful for detection when a soft tissue component is present.
6. Compared with the location of uncomplicated Paget's disease, these sarcomas have a predilection for the humerus and only rarely arise in the spine.

## ■ Radiographic Differential Diagnosis

1. Paget's disease with marked lysis.
2. Florid Paget's disease extending into soft tissues.

## ■ Pathologic Features

*Gross*

1. A destructive lesion involves the bone and extends into the soft tissues.
2. The soft, fleshy tumor generally is whitish to brown in color.

*Microscopic*

1. At low magnification the tumor is highly cellular.
2. The tumor generally is composed of spindle cells.
3. At higher magnification, the spindle cells show significant pleomorphism and cytologic atypia.
4. The specific diagnosis may be that of osteosarcoma, fibrosarcoma, or malignant fibrous histiocytoma.

■ **Pathologic Differential Diagnosis**

Benign lesions:
1. Lytic phase of Paget's disease (radiographic, primarily).
2. Fracture callus.
3. Myositis ossificans (heterotopic ossification).

Malignant lesions:
1. Malignant lymphoma.
2. Osteosarcoma.
3. Fibrosarcoma.
4. Malignant fibrous histiocytoma.

■ **Treatment**

**Primary Modality:** Usually the tumor's aggressive behavior, with extensive local involvement, requires amputation to achieve an adequately wide surgical margin.

**Other Possible Approaches:** preoperative chemotherapy and limb-saving resection if surgical staging suggests that an adequately wide margin can be achieved. Radiation therapy is used for surgically inaccessible lesions, and aggressive approach with thoracotomy is employed for pulmonary metastases.

### References

Haibach H, Farrell C, and Dittrich FJ: Neoplasms arising in Paget's disease of bone: a study of 82 cases. Am J Clin Pathol 83:594–600, 1985.

Wick MR, Siegal GP, McLeod RA, et al: Sarcomas of bone complicating osteitis deformans (Paget's disease): fifty years' experience. Am J Surg Pathol 5:47–59, 1981.

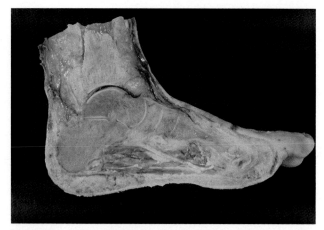

**Figure 37–1.** This gross specimen shows a case of Paget's sarcoma involving the distal tibia. The patient initially had suffered a pathologic fracture of the distal tibia and been treated conservatively for the fracture, as the underlying malignancy was radiographically subtle. The tumor has broken through the cortex and extended into the soft tissues of the foot.

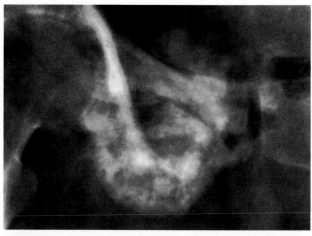

**Figure 37–3.** A blastic Paget's sarcoma, arising in the ischium and pubis in a region of pre-existing Paget's disease, is shown in this radiograph. The soft tissue component of the tumor contains bony mineralization indicative of an osteosarcoma.

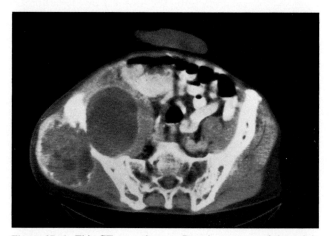

**Figure 37–4.** This CT scan shows a Paget's sarcoma of the pelvis with a large soft tissue component surrounding the iliac bone. Both innominate bones show evidence of Paget's disease as well.

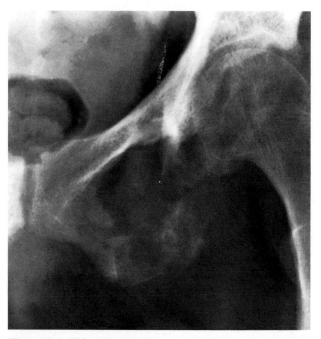

**Figure 37–2.** This radiograph shows a lytic Paget's sarcoma arising in the ischium with pre-existing Paget's disease and causing considerable bone destruction.

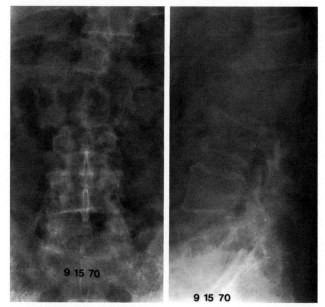

**Figure 37–5:** This radiograph reveals extensive lysis of a vertebra due to uncomplicated Paget's disease. The radiographic appearance is that of a malignancy; however, the spine is a rare site for this complication of Paget's disease.

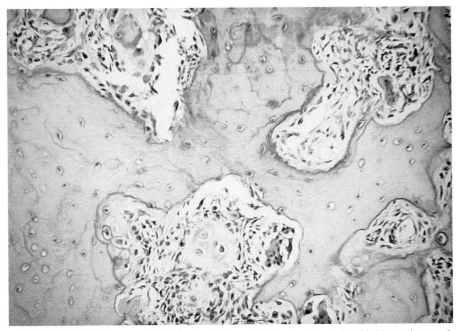

**Figure 37–6.** Paget's sarcomas may show a variety of histologic patterns. As this photomicrograph illustrates, osteosarcoma is the most common.

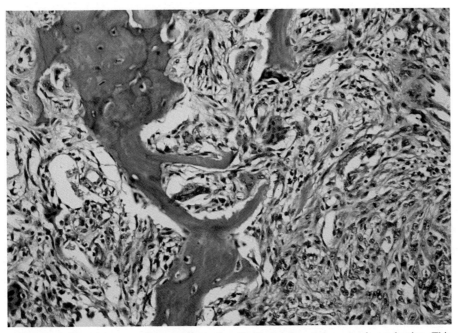

**Figure 37–7.** Some sarcomas that complicate Paget's disease do not show matrix production. This photomicrograph shows such a case. These lesions may be classified as fibrosarcomas or as malignant fibrous histiocytomas, depending upon other features evident in the tumor.

# CHAPTER 38

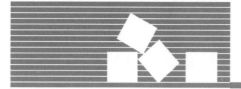

# Postradiation Sarcoma

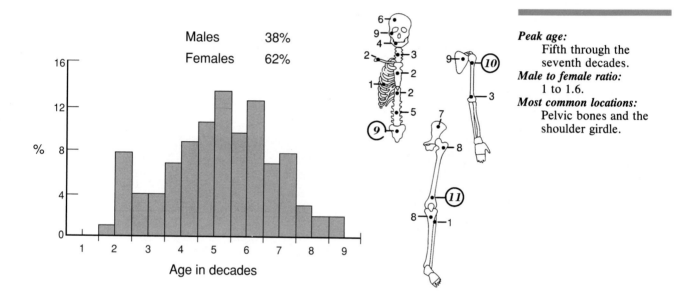

Males 38%
Females 62%

% (y-axis: 0, 4, 8, 12, 16)

Age in decades (x-axis: 1 through 9)

*Peak age:*
    Fifth through the
    seventh decades.
*Male to female ratio:*
    1 to 1.6.
*Most common locations:*
    Pelvic bones and the
    shoulder girdle.

■ **Clinical Symptoms**

1. Pain is felt in the region of prior radiation.
2. The interval between radiation therapy and diagnosis of sarcoma has varied from 2.75 to 55 years in cases treated at the Mayo Clinic, with an average interval of 15.1 years.
3. A swelling may be noted by the patient.

■ **Clinical Signs**

1. A tender mass lesion is found on physical examination.
2. Skin changes compatible with prior radiation therapy may be present.

■ **Major Radiographic Features**

1. The tumor may arise from normal bone or in an area of a pre-existing lesion within the radiation portal.

2. The underlying bone often is altered by radiation, surgery, the pre-existing abnormality, or some combination of these.
3. The underlying changes in the affected bone may obscure the lesion early in the course of the disease.
4. The latent period ranges from 2.75 to 55 years, with an average of 15 years.
5. Postradiation sarcomas are similar to conventional tumors radiographically.
6. A soft tissue mass, cortical destruction, and extraosseous bone production are indicative of sarcoma.

■ **Radiographic Differential Diagnosis**

1. Metastatic disease.
2. Radiation change without sarcoma.
3. Osteoporosis.
4. Insufficiency stress fracture.

226

## ■ Pathologic Features

### Gross

1. These tumors tend to be soft and fleshy.
2. The tumor has most commonly extended beyond the confines of the affected bone and has an associated soft tissue mass.
3. Foci of hemorrhage and necrosis may be identifiable.
4. Matrix production in the form of osteoid or even cartilage may be seen, and calcification may be present on a degenerative basis.

### Microscopic

1. At low magnification the pattern varies from tumor to tumor. Of 103 postradiation sarcomas compiled by the Mayo Clinic, the majority (51 per cent) showed osteoid production and were classified as osteosarcomas.
2. Spindle cell tumors lacking osteoid matrix production were the second largest group, accounting for 42 per cent of the total, with the majority of these being classified as fibrosarcomas and the remainder as malignant fibrous histiocytomas.
3. At higher magnification the cytologic characteristics are those of a pleomorphic high-grade sarcoma. The nuclei vary in size, shape, and nuclear staining characteristics.

## ■ Pathologic Differential Diagnosis

Benign lesions:
1. Reactive spindle cell proliferation in the region of prior radiation.
2. Fracture callus at a site of pathologic fracture after radiation therapy.

Malignant lesions:
1. Osteosarcoma.
2. Fibrosarcoma.
3. Malignant fibrous histiocytoma.

## ■ Treatment

**Primary Modality:** preoperative chemotherapy and limb-saving resection if a wide surgical margin can be achieved. Reconstruction is individualized and depends on the location of the tumor. Amputation will be necessary if surgical staging indicates that an adequately wide margin cannot be achieved to preserve the neurovascular structures.

**Other Possible Approaches:** radiation therapy for lesions in inaccessible sites, thoracotomy for pulmonary metastases, or chemotherapy protocols similar to those used for osteosarcoma.

### References

Weatherby RP, Dahlin DC, and Ivins JC: Postradiation sarcoma of bone: review of 78 Mayo Clinic cases. Mayo Clin Proc 56:294–306, 1981.

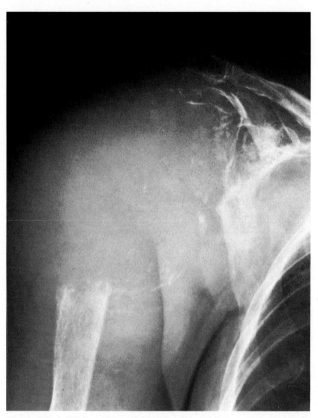

**Figure 38–1.** This radiograph shows a postradiation sarcoma of the proximal humerus, with nearly complete destruction of the bone and an associated soft tissue mass. The tumor arose eight years after radiation therapy for carcinoma of the breast. Radiation changes are present in the remaining humerus and the scapula.

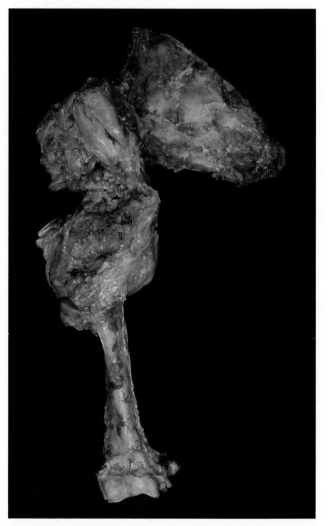

**Figure 38–2.** The specimen from the forequarter amputation performed in the case shown in Figure 38–1 shows the total destruction of the proximal humerus. Hemorrhagic necrosis and soft tissue extension are commonly seen in postradiation sarcomas of this size.

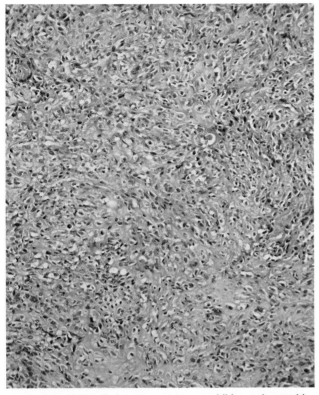

**Figure 38–3.** Postradiation sarcomas may exhibit nearly any histologic pattern of growth and differentiation. This tumor, which arose in the distal femur of a young woman who had received radiation therapy for a hemangioendothelial sarcoma, shows bony matrix production.

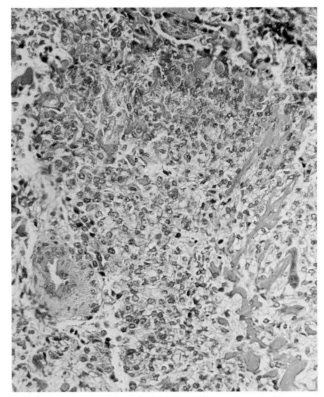

**Figure 38–5.** This photomicrograph shows a postradiation osteosarcoma that arose after treatment for histiocytosis X of the mandible.

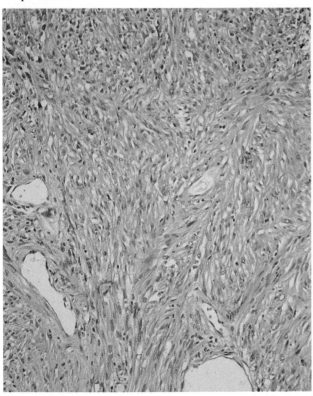

**Figure 38–4.** This purely spindle cell sarcoma lacked evidence of matrix production and was classified as a postradiation fibrosarcoma. The tumor arose in the humerus 55 years after radiation therapy.

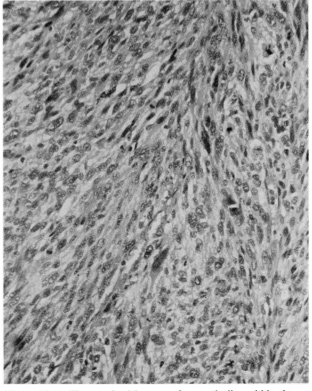

**Figure 38–6.** The proximal humerus frequently lies within the radiation port for patients receiving adjuvant radiation therapy for metastatic breast carcinoma. This fibrosarcoma arose in the proximal humerus in such a clinical setting.

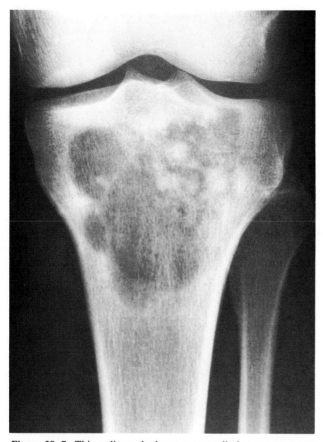

**Figure 38–7.** This radiograph shows a postradiation osteosarcoma of the proximal tibia. The large, malignant-appearing tumor shows areas of ossification.

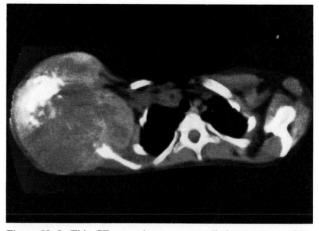

**Figure 38–8.** This CT scan shows a postradiation sarcoma of the proximal humerus. The ossified malignancy also demonstrates a huge, necrotic soft tissue component.

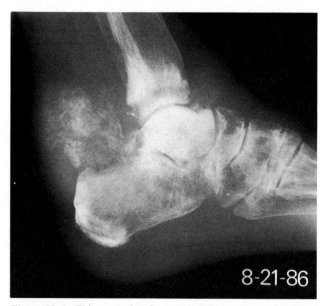

**Figure 38–9.** This example of a postradiation sarcoma developed multifocally in the foot and ankle of a radium watch–dial painter.

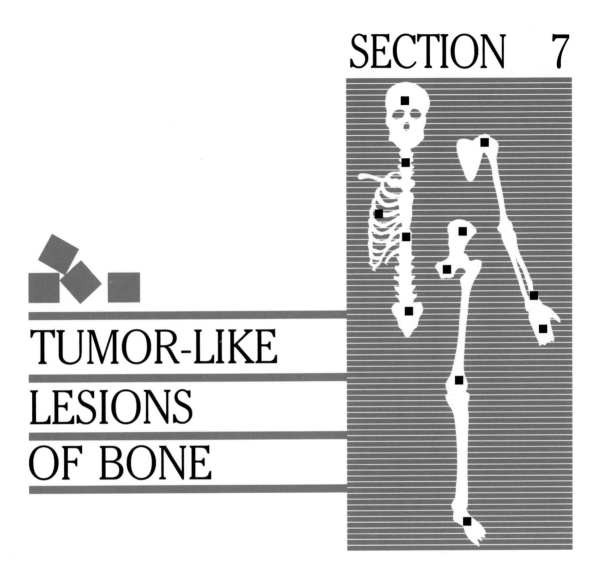

# SECTION 7

# TUMOR-LIKE LESIONS OF BONE

# CHAPTER 39

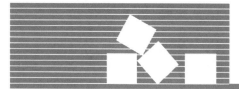

# Aneurysmal Bone Cyst

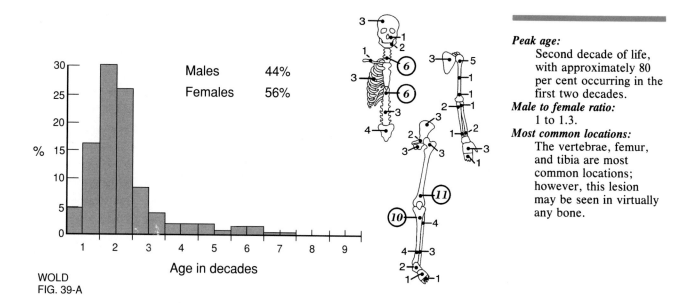

Males 44%

Females 56%

WOLD
FIG. 39-A

**Peak age:**
Second decade of life, with approximately 80 per cent occurring in the first two decades.
**Male to female ratio:**
1 to 1.3.
**Most common locations:**
The vertebrae, femur, and tibia are most common locations; however, this lesion may be seen in virtually any bone.

■ **Clinical Symptoms**

1. Pain is the most common symptom at presentation; it is usually of short duration.
2. Swelling may be noticed, and the size of the lesion tends to increase until therapy is instituted.

■ **Clinical Signs**

1. Swelling may be evident on physical examination.
2. Aneurysmal bone cyst frequently involves the vertebra—usually the posterior elements—and as such may cause signs and symptoms of cord compression or compression of emerging nerves.

■ **Major Radiographic Features**

1. "Ballooned" or "aneurysmal" cystic expansion of the affected bone is evident.

2. No significant matrix mineralization is seen.
3. The lesion affects the metaphysis in long bones and the dorsal elements in vertebral locations.
4. Sclerotic rim and periosteal new bone formation are common.
5. The tumor may have an aggressive appearance, simulating that of a sarcoma.

■ **Radiographic Differential Diagnosis**

1. Unicameral bone cyst (simple cyst).
2. Giant cell tumor.
3. Sarcoma, particularly osteosarcoma, telangiectatic type.
4. Osteoblastoma when in the vertebra.

■ **Pathologic Features**

*Gross*

1. The lesional tissue is hemorrhagic, consisting of

unclotted blood and more "fleshy," solid aggregates of tissue.
2. Blood may fill the region of the tumor as the overlying bone is unroofed, but it does not spurt in a pulsatile fashion from the lesion.
3. At the periphery of the lesion an "eggshell"-thin layer of periosteal new bone is characteristically present.

### Microscopic

1. With low magnification, cavernous spaces that may be filled with blood are identified.
2. The walls of the spaces contain spindled fibroblastic cells, multinucleated giant cells, and thin strands of bone.
3. With high magnification the spaces are seen to lack an endothelial lining.

### ■ Pathologic Differential Diagnosis

Benign lesions:
1. Giant cell tumor.
2. Giant cell reparative granuloma (giant cell reaction).
3. Simple bone cyst.

Malignant lesions:
1. Telangiectatic osteosarcoma.

### ■ Treatment

**Primary Modality:** excision, curettage, and bone grafting. When the lesion is in an expendable bone such as the fibula or a rib, resection with a marginal or wide margin is preferred. In a patient who is asymptomatic, persistence of a cyst in a portion of a grafted lesion that has not been expanding on serial roentgenograms may be managed by close observation.

**Other Possible Approaches:** surgical adjuvant treatment with cryosurgery or chemical cautery. Radiation is not recommended because of the potential for malignant transformation.

### References

Dahlin DC, and McLeod RA: Aneurysmal bone cyst and other nonneoplastic conditions. Skeletal Radiol 8:243–250, 1982.

Levy WM, Miller AS, Bonakdarpour A, and Aegerter W: Aneurysmal bone cyst secondary to other osseous lesions: report of 57 cases. Am J Clin Pathol 63:1–8, 1975.

Ruiter DJ, vanRijssel TG, and ven der Velde EA: Aneurysmal bone cysts: A clinicopathological study of 105 cases. Cancer 39:2231–2239, 1977.

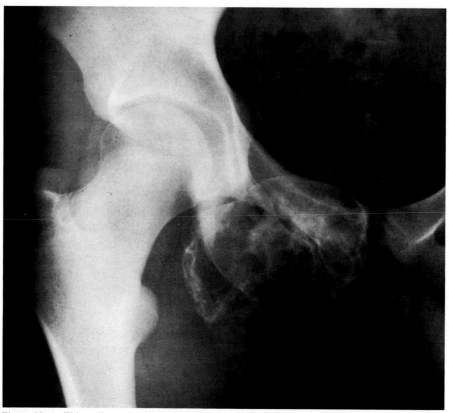

**Figure 39–1.** This radiograph of the pelvis shows a large aneurysmal bone cyst of the ischium and pubis, with marked expansion of the affected bones. No matrix mineralization is present, and the lesion is surrounded by a thin shell of bone.

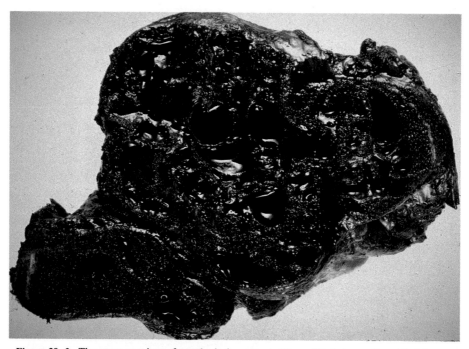

**Figure 39–2.** The gross specimen from the lesion seen in Figure 39–1 shows the typical features of aneurysmal bone cyst. The lesion is hemorrhagic and cystic. Numerous septa are identified; they may be somewhat gritty, as bone may be present in them.

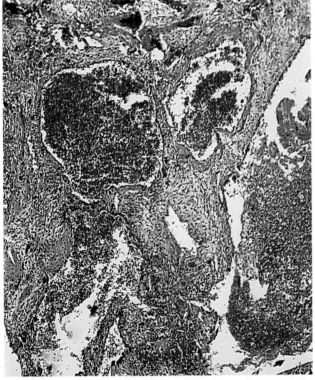

**Figure 39–3.** At low magnification aneurysmal bone cysts generally contain numerous blood-filled spaces, as is illustrated in this photomicrograph.

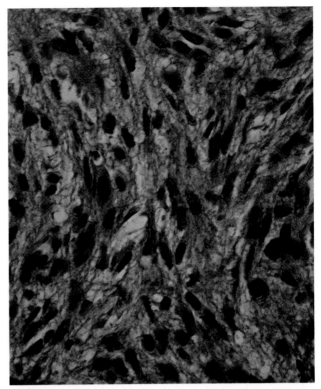

**Figure 39–5.** At higher magnification, the solid portions of aneurysmal bone cyst show a loose arrangement of the spindle cells. Mitotic activity may be brisk, this being the histologic counterpart of the clinical fact that the lesion may grow rapidly.

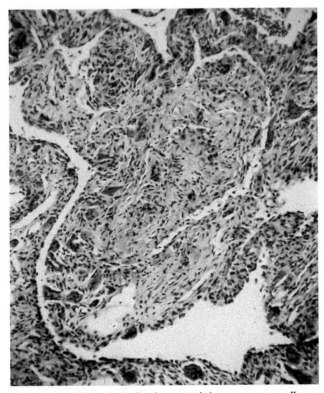

**Figure 39–4.** When the lesion is curetted the spaces may collapse, as this photomicrograph shows. Blood may not be prominent since it may be lost during processing of the specimen. When the curetted specimen is collapsed, the presence of benign multinucleated giant cells within the lesion may result in a histologic pattern superficially mimicking that of giant cell tumor.

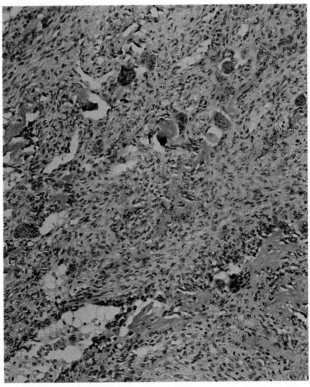

**Figure 39–6.** The solid portion of this aneurysmal bone cyst of the tibia shows bone production. This, combined with the aggressive radiographic appearance that may be present and the brisk mitotic activity generally seen in such lesions, may lead to a mistaken diagnosis of osteosarcoma.

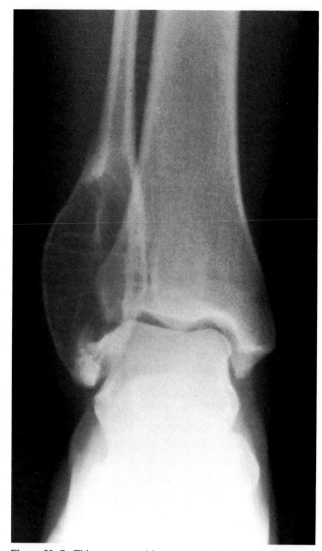

**Figure 39–7.** This aneurysmal bone cyst of the lower fibula shows marked expansion of the metaphysis. The overall appearance is that of a benign process.

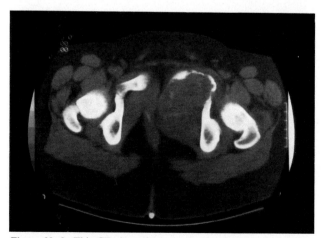

**Figure 39–8.** This CT view of a large aneurysmal bone cyst of the pelvis shows an inhomogeneous soft tissue component associated with the lesion. Such an appearance may suggest a diagnosis of sarcoma.

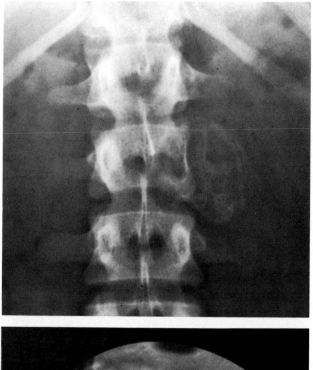

A

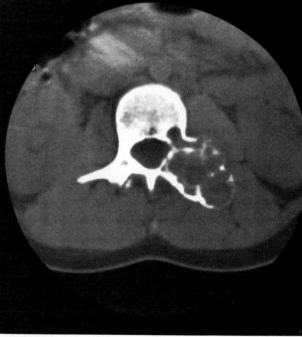

B

**Figure 39–9.** This radiograph (*A*) and CT scan (*B*) demonstrate an aneurysmal bone cyst involving the L2 vertebra. When the vertebrae are involved, it is generally the posterior or dorsal elements that are affected; the radiographic appearance is that of an expansile, lytic defect.

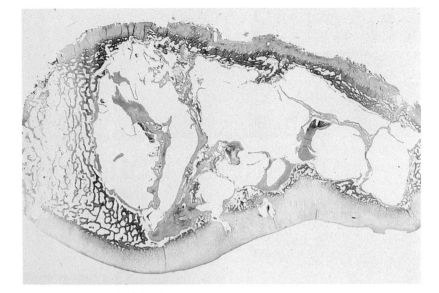

**Figure 39–10.** Multiple septa are present in an aneurysmal bone cyst, as is shown in this low-power photomicrograph in which the fibrous septa are seen traversing the cystic space.

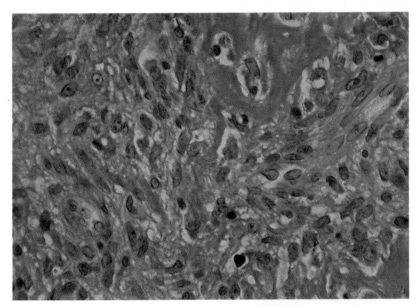

**Figure 39–11.** The fibrous bone present in the septa of the lesion may suggest the possibility that the lesion is an osteosarcoma. However, the loose arrangement of the lesion, its vascular appearance, and the presence of bone may also mimic the appearance of osteoblastoma.

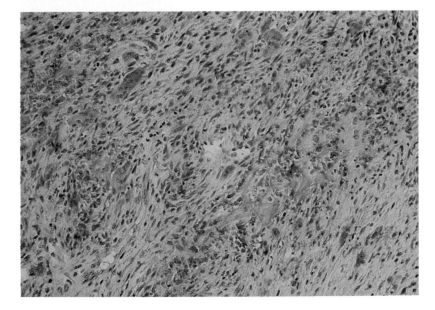

**Figure 39–12.** The loose pattern of arrangement shown in this low-power photomicrograph indicates that the lesion is proliferative in nature and not neoplastic.

# CHAPTER 40

## Unicameral Bone Cyst (Simple Cyst)

*Peak age:*
First two decades of life.
*Male to female ratio:*
Approximately 1 to 1.
*Most common locations:*
Proximal humerus, proximal femur, and proximal tibia.

■ **Clinical Symptoms**

1. The majority of tumors are asymptomatic.
2. Onset of pain is abrupt (associated with pathologic fracture).
3. Rarely, swelling in the region of the lesion may be noticed.

■ **Clinical Signs**

1. The majority of these lesions are incidental radiographic "abnormalities."
2. A painful mass occasionally may be identified on physical examination.

■ **Major Radiographic Features**

1. Cysts usually occur in the upper humerus or upper femur.
2. They frequently abut the epiphyseal plate.
3. They are often large and elongated.
4. Expansion is usually present but does not exceed the width of the epiphyseal plate.

5. There is sharp margination, often with trabeculation.
6. Pathologic fracture occurs and may result in healing or bone fragment settling to the dependent part of the lesion, indicative of fluid.

■ **Radiographic Differential Diagnosis**

1. Aneurysmal bone cyst.
2. Fibrous dysplasia.

■ **Pathologic Features**

*Gross*

1. The cystic cavity usually contains a straw-colored fluid.
2. If there has been bleeding into the cyst, pathologic fracture, or a previous attempt to needle the lesion, the fluid may be blood-tinged or frankly bloody.
3. Occasionally, partial or complete septation of the cyst may be seen.

*Microscopic*

1. At low magnification the lining of the cyst appears as a thin rim of fibrous connective tissue.
2. Thicker areas of the cyst wall contain multinucleated giant cells.
3. Amorphous eosinophilic debris (probably fibrin) frequently is identified in the hypocellular fibrous connective tissue. This may undergo calcification, resulting in an appearance simulating that of cementum.
4. At higher magnification no cytologic atypia is appreciated.

## ■ Pathologic Differential Diagnosis

Benign lesions:
1. Aneurysmal bone cyst.
2. Giant cell tumor.

Malignant lesions:
1. Rarely, an osteosarcoma has been mistakenly treated as a simple cyst. Radiographic features should aid in avoiding this mistake.

## ■ Treatment

**Primary Modality:** dual-needle aspiration of the cyst and injection of methylprednisolone. Multiple steroid injections may be necessary to promote healing of the cyst.

**Other Possible Approaches:** In patients with loss of structural integrity in a weight-bearing bone associated with a large cyst, curettage and grafting are indicated.

## References

Bauer TW, and Dorfman HD: Intraosseous ganglion: a clinicopathologic study of 11 cases. Am J Surg Pathol 6:207–213, 1982.

Boseker EH, Bickel WH, and Dahlin DC: A clinicopathologic study of simple unicameral bone cysts. Surg Gynecol Obstet *127*:550–560, 1968.

Capanna R, Dal Monte A, Gitelis S, and Campanacci M: The natural history of unicameral bone cyst after steroid injection. Clin Orthop *166*:204–211, 1982.

Schajowicz F, Sainz MC, and Slullitel JA: Juxta-articular bone cysts (intra-osseous ganglia): a clinicopathological study of eighty-eight cases. J Bone Joint Surg *61B*:107–116, 1979.

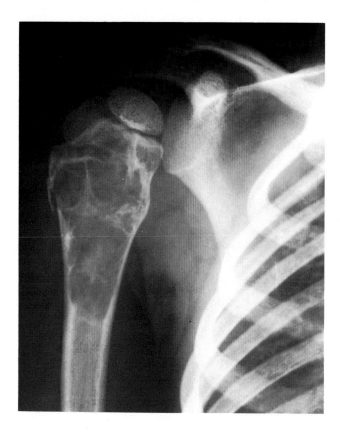

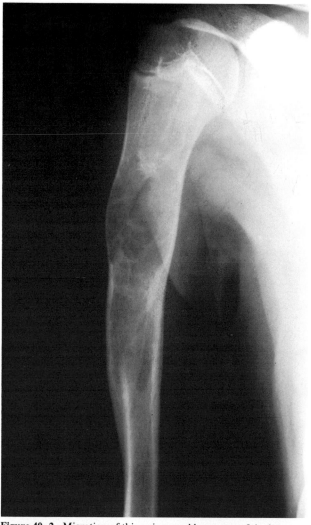

**Figure 40–1.** This radiograph shows a unicameral bone cyst abutting against the physis of the upper humerus. The lesion has resulted in mild expansion of the bone and shows sharp margination. A pathologic fracture is present, and trabeculation is evident.

**Figure 40–2.** Migration of this unicameral bone cyst of the humerus has resulted in a diaphyseal location for the lesion.

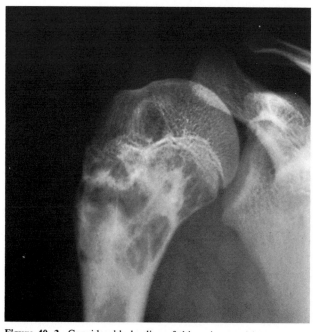

**Figure 40–3.** Considerable healing of this unicameral bone cyst of the proximal humerus has occurred after a pathologic fracture sustained eight months earlier.

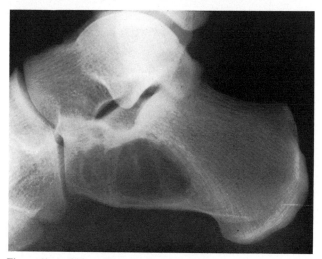

**Figure 40–4.** This radiograph shows a simple cyst of the calcaneus.

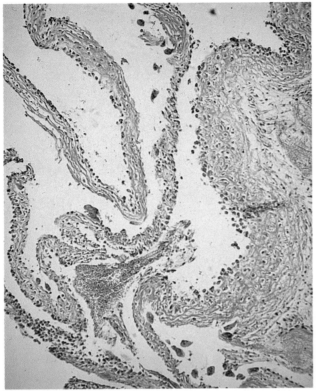

**Figure 40-5.** At low magnification, curretted fragments of tissue from a simple cyst may show septa similar to those seen in aneurysmal bone cyst. Usually they show only a thin lining on the bone.

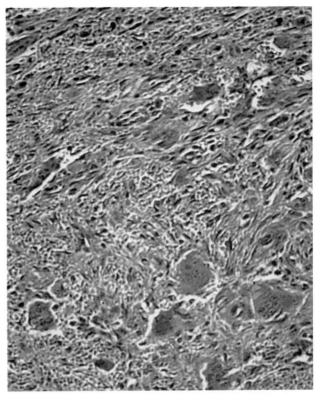

**Figure 40-7.** Some regions of the wall may contain multinucleated giant cell and have histologic features identical with aneurysmal bone cyst.

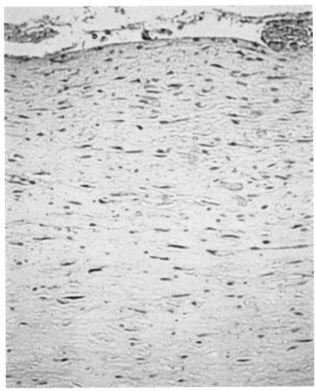

**Figure 40-6.** At higher magnification, the wall of the cyst is composed of hypocellular connective tissue with bland cytologic features.

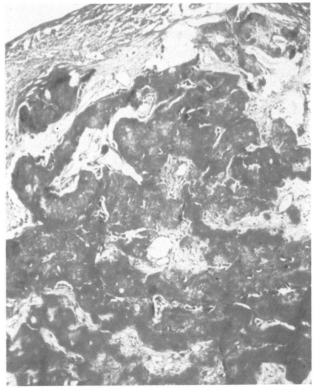

**Figure 40-8.** Eosinophilic aggregates of calcified fibrinous debris may be identified in the wall of the cyst. The histologic features of such debris may resemble cementum.

# CHAPTER 41

# Giant Cell Reaction (Giant Cell Reparative Granuloma)

*Peak age:*
  Adulthood.
*Male to female ratio:*
  Approximately 1 to 1.
*Most common location:*
  Small bones of the hands and feet.

■ **Clinical Symptoms**

1. Approximately 50 per cent of patients present with local pain as their primary complaint.
2. Approximately 50 per cent of patients present with a localized swelling.
3. Rarely the lesion is asymptomatic and incidentally discovered on radiographic examination.

■ **Clinical Signs**

1. A mass lesion may be discovered on physical examination.
2. The mass may be tender to palpation.
3. There are no findings on physical examination in many cases.

■ **Major Radiographic Features**

1. Most lesions are purely lytic although occasional sclerosis or calcification is seen.
2. Expansion and cortical thinning as well as sharp margination are invariably seen.
3. Cortical breakthrough and periosteal new bone are occasionally seen.
4. Most lesions extend to the end of the bone after epiphyseal closure.

■ **Radiographic Differential Diagnosis**

1. Aneurysmal bone cyst.
2. Giant cell tumor.
3. Enchondroma.

## ■ Pathologic Features

### Gross

1. Curetted fragments of bone are reddish-brown in color.
2. In contrast to aneurysmal bone cyst, the volume of tissue curetted approximates the size of the lesion as identified radiographically.

### Microscopic

1. At low magnification the lesional tissue is composed of spindle cells lying in a fibrous stroma.
2. Numerous multinucleated giant cells are present; these tend to be arranged in a vaguely clustered manner.
3. Reactive new bone with prominent osteoblastic activity resembling osteoblastoma is present.
4. At higher magnification, the mononuclear stromal cells and the giant cells lack cytologic atypia.
5. Mitotic figures may be identified but in general the mitotic rate is low.

## ■ Pathologic Differential Diagnosis

Benign lesions:

1. Aneurysmal bone cyst.
2. Brown tumor of hyperparathyroidism.
3. Giant cell tumor.
4. Fracture callus.

Malignant lesions:

1. Malignant fibrous histiocytoma.
2. Osteosarcoma.

## ■ Treatment

**Primary Modality:** Excision by curettage and bone grafting as necessary are usually adequate.

**Other Possible Approaches:** en bloc resection and skeletal reconstruction when this can be performed without significant compromise in function.

## References

Averill RM, Smith RJ, and Campbell CJ: Giant-cell tumors of the bones of the hand. J Hand Surg 5:39–50, 1980.

D'Alonzo RT, Pitcock JA, and Milford LW: Giant-cell reaction of bone: report of two cases. J Bone Joint Surg 54A:1267–1271, 1972.

Glass TA, Mills SE, Fechner RE, et al: Giant-cell reparative granuloma of the hands and feet. Radiology 149:65–68, 1983.

Lorenzo JC, and Dorfman HD: Giant-cell reparative granuloma of short tubular bones of the hands and feet. Am J Surg Pathol 4:551–563, 1980.

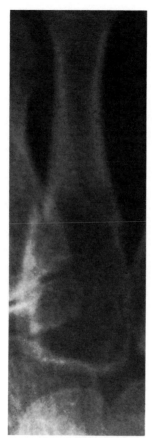

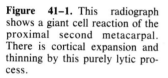

**Figure 41–1.** This radiograph shows a giant cell reaction of the proximal second metacarpal. There is cortical expansion and thinning by this purely lytic process.

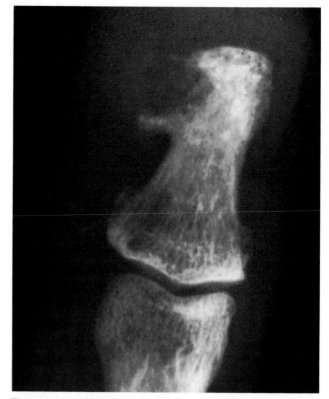

**Figure 41–2.** A giant cell reaction of the distal phalanx is shown in this radiograph. The lesion arose eccentrically and has extended into the soft tissues.

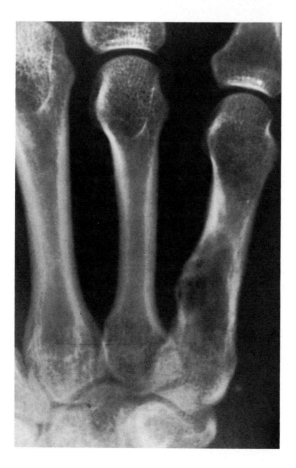

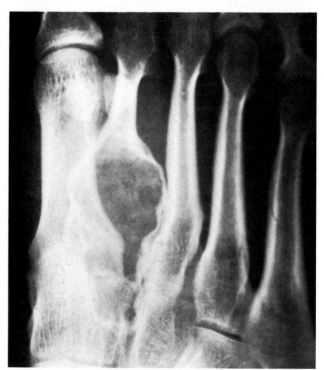

**Figure 41–4.** Marked bony expansion has resulted from the presence of this large, lytic giant cell reaction of the proximal second metatarsal.

**Figure 41–3.** In this purely lytic giant cell reaction of the proximal metacarpal, the lesion is well marginated and shows cortical expansion and thinning.

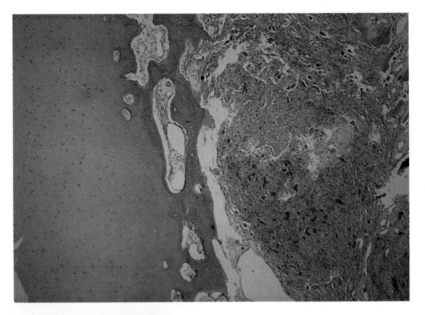

**Figure 41–5.** This photomicrograph shows a giant cell reaction extending to the end of a small bone in the hand. At low magnification, giant cells may be seen to slightly cluster in these lesions.

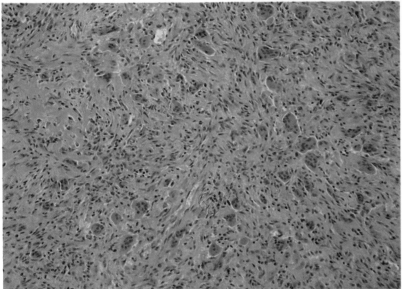

**Figure 41–6.** Giant cell reactions show a distinctly spindled mononuclear stromal component, as this photomicrograph illustrates. This is in contrast with benign giant cell tumors, in which the mononuclear stromal component is round to oval in shape.

**Figure 41–7.** The stromal component of giant cell reactions is generally more collagenous than that of giant cell tumors. Osteoid may be seen in the stroma as well.

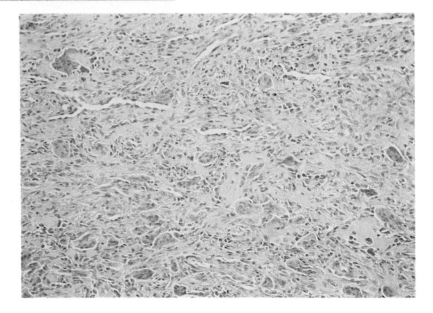

# CHAPTER 42

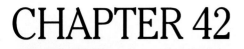

# Fibroma (Metaphyseal Fibrous Defect)

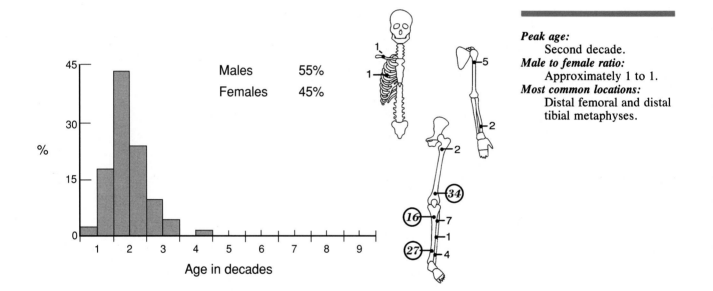

Males 55%
Females 45%

45

30

15

0

%

1  2  3  4  5  6  7  8  9
Age in decades

*Peak age:*
Second decade.
*Male to female ratio:*
Approximately 1 to 1.
*Most common locations:*
Distal femoral and distal tibial metaphyses.

■ **Clinical Symptoms**

1. These lesions are usually asymptomatic and are discovered on radiographic examination for an unrelated condition.
2. Local pain of short duration may be present.
3. Pathologic fracture may be the first clinical symptom.

■ **Clinical Signs**

1. Physical examination is usually unrevealing in these cases.
2. A slight swelling may be present if the affected bone is near the skin, e.g., the distal tibia.

■ **Major Radiographic Features**

1. The lesion is metaphyseal in location.
2. The lesion is expansile and sharply marginated and located in the cortex.
3. The lesion appears multilocular and has a scalloped margin.
4. The long axis of the lesion generally parallels that of the affected bone, and there is a sclerotic rim surrounding it.
5. Multiple lesions may be present.

■ **Radiographic Differential Diagnosis**

1. Chondromyxoid fibroma.
2. Fibrous dysplasia.

246

3. Histiocytosis X (Langerhans' cell granulomatosis).

## ■ Pathologic Features

### Gross

1. The cortex may be attenuated in the area of the lesion but remains intact unless pathologic fracture has occurred.
2. The lesion is well demarcated from the surrounding bone.
3. Curetted fragments are fibrous and vary in color from yellow to brown, depending on the proportion of fibrous tissue to lipid-laden or hemosiderin-laden histiocytes present in the lesion.

### Microscopic

1. At low magnification the pattern is variable from region to region. Zones of spindle cells are arranged in a storiform pattern and interspersed with other foci containing more abundant histiocytic cells.
2. Giant cells are scattered throughout the lesion in irregular clusters (in general these cells contain fewer nuclei than the giant cells of giant cell tumor).
3. Clusters of lipophages are scattered irregularly throughout the lesion.
4. Clusters of hemosiderin-laden macrophages are similarly dispersed.
5. On higher magnification the nuclei of the spindled cells and histiocytes are regular. Mitotic figures may be present.
6. When pathologic fracture occurs, there may be associated reactive new bone formation.

## ■ Pathologic Differential Diagnosis

Benign lesions:
1. Giant cell tumor.
2. Benign fibrous histiocytoma.
3. Giant cell tumor of tendon sheath type.
4. Pigmented villonodular synovitis.

Malignant lesions:
1. Malignant fibrous histiocytoma.
2. Osteosarcoma (if pathologic fracture and reactive new bone are misinterpreted).

## ■ Treatment

**Primary Modality:** If the diagnosis is certain and the lesion does not threaten the strength of the bone, observation alone is indicated.

**Other Possible Approaches:** Large lesions occupying more than 50 per cent of the bone diameter pose the risk of fracture. Curettage and bone grafting are curative. Pathologic fractures should be allowed to heal prior to surgical intervention.

## Reference

Steiner GC: Fibrous cortical defect and nonossifying fibroma of bone: a study of the ultrastructure. Arch Pathol 97:205–210, 1974.

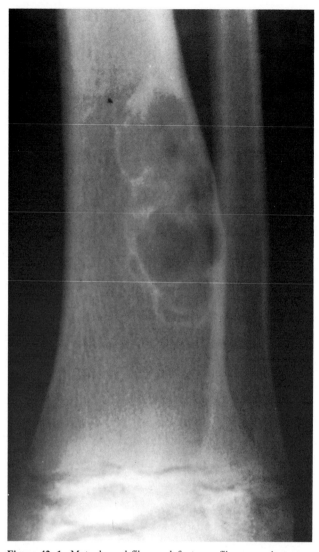

**Figure 42–1.** Metaphyseal fibrous defects, or fibromas, characteristically have a sharp peripheral margin and a sclerotic rim. These
features are well demonstrated in this lesion of the distal diametaphyseal region of the tibia. The affected bone may be expanded, as
in this case, and the lesion characteristically has a scalloped margin.

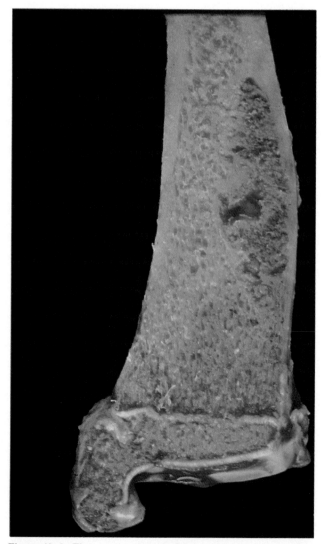

**Figure 42–2.** The gross pathologic features in this case correlate
closely with the radiographic features shown in Figure 42–1. The
patient had an incidental fibroma identified at the time of diagnosis
of a distal femoral osteosarcoma, for which an above-the-knee amputation was performed.

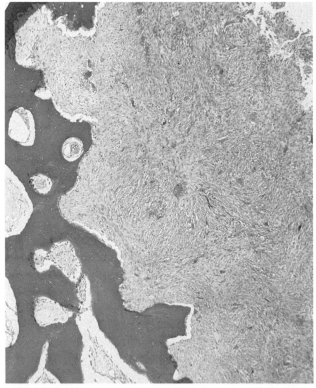

**Figure 42–3.** At low magnification, the well-circumscribed nature of a metaphyseal fibrous defect is evident at the periphery of the lesion. This photomicrograph shows the edge of a fibular lesion.

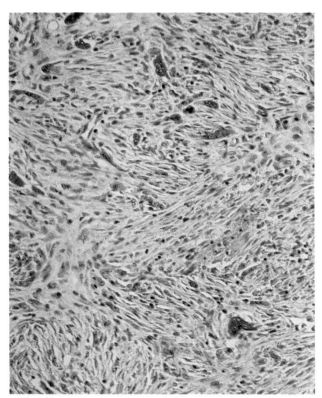

**Figure 42–5.** The pattern of arrangement of the cell at low magnification is frequently storiform, as is shown in this field from a proximal tibial lesion.

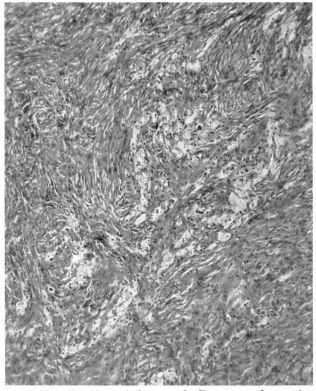

**Figure 42–4.** The histologic features of a fibroma vary from region to region within the lesion. The cells vary in shape from spindled to round; some show phagocytic activity resulting in hemosiderin-laden or lipid-laden cytoplasm, as is illustrated in this photomicrograph.

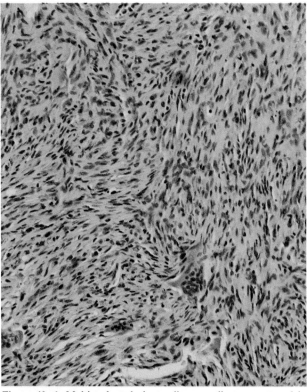

**Figure 42–6.** Multinucleated giant cells generally are scattered in the lesion; however, they may cluster slightly. This feature may suggest the histologic diagnosis of giant cell tumor; however, the location, radiographic features, age, and spindled nature of the stromal cells are all characteristics that militate against such a diagnosis.

**Figure 42–8.** This fibroma of the distal fibula also shows the sharp margination and peripheral sclerosis characteristic of this group of lesions.

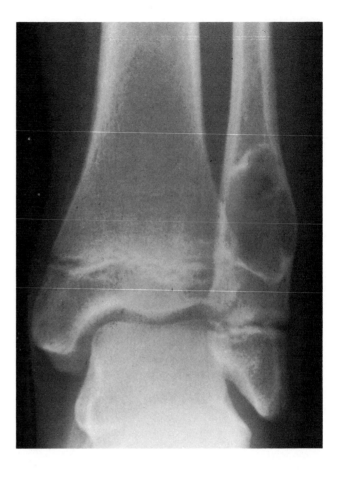

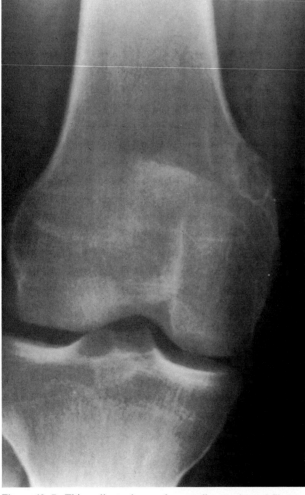

**Figure 42–7.** This radiograph reveals a small metaphyseal fibroma with a sharp sclerotic margin and slight expansion involving the distal femur. Such a lesion can be confidently identified on the basis of the radiographic features, and surgical intervention is unnecessary.

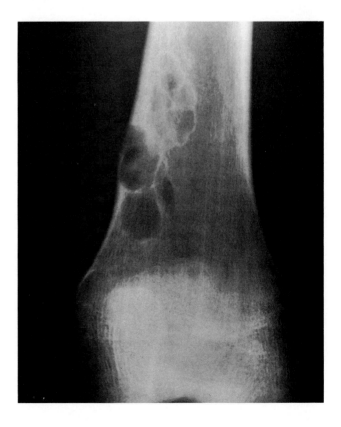

**Figure 42–9.** This radiograph illustrates the multilocular appearance of a fibroma involving the distal femur.

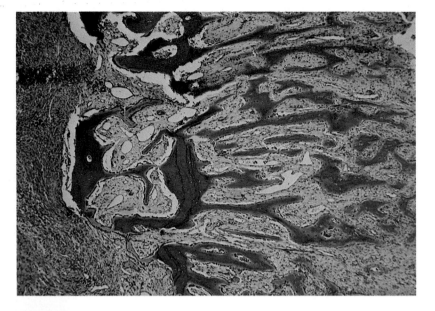

**Figure 42–10.** If pathologic fracture has occurred through a fibroma, a prominent periosteal reaction may be present. Although the orderly arrangement of the reaction at low magnification is a clue to its benign nature, disregarding this feature may result in a mistaken diagnosis of malignancy based upon the mitotic activity and production of osteoid that are evident at high magnification.

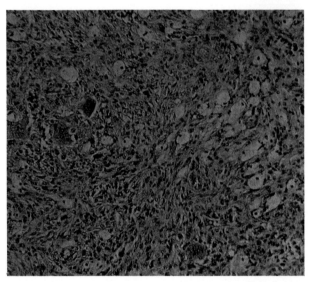

**Figure 42–11.** Fibroma and benign fibrous histiocytoma share histologic features; both lesions show phagocytic activity and a storiform pattern of growth. The diagnosis of benign fibrous histiocytoma is only viable in a clinical setting in which fibroma is rare. This fibroma shows the characteristic histologic features of these two lesions.

**Figure 42–12.** Numerous multinucleated giant cells may be present in a fibroma, as in this case involving the proximal tibia.

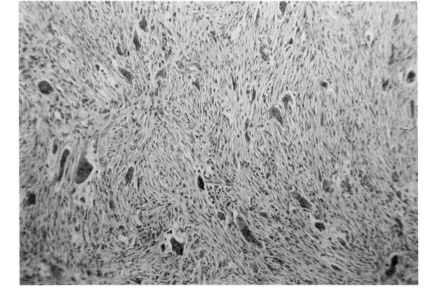

# CHAPTER 43

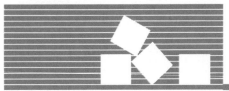

# Avulsive Cortical Irregularity (Fibrous Cortical Defect, Periosteal Desmoid)

***Peak age:***
Second decade.
***Male to female ratio:***
Approximately 1 to 1.
***Most common location:***
Almost exclusively found on the posteromedial aspect of the distal femur, in relation to the insertion of the adductor magnus muscle.

■ **Clinical Symptoms**

1. These lesions are invariably silent clinically.
2. They are discovered as incidental radiographic findings, often following some trauma.

■ **Clinical Signs**

1. There are no findings on physical examination.

■ **Major Radiographic Features**

1. The lesion is characteristically located along medial posterior supracondylar ridges 1 to 2 cm above the epiphyseal plate, best seen in external rotation.
2. There is cortical fuzziness, irregularity, or spiculation.
3. There may be a small cortical defect.
4. There is no soft tissue mass.
5. It is usually found in boys (3:1), and a third are bilateral.

■ **Radiographic Differential Diagnosis**

1. Osteosarcoma.

■ **Pathologic Features**

*Gross*

1. In general, these lesions are identified radiographically; biopsy is not necessary.

2. If biopsied, the lesional tissue is nondescript, fibrous, and soft.

*Microscopic*

1. At low magnification the lesion is composed of spindle cells.
2. Lesional tissue is hypocellular, and abundant collagen is produced by the spindle-cell component of the lesion.
3. At higher magnification the fibroblasts show no cytologic atypia.
4. Mitotic figures are not identified.

■ **Pathologic Differential Diagnosis**

Benign lesions:
1. Fibroma.
2. Fibromatosis.
Malignant lesions:
1. Fibrosarcoma, well differentiated.

■ **Treatment**

**Primary Modality:** If the radiographic features are classic, no therapy need be initiated.
**Other Possible Approaches:** If the radiographic features are sufficiently atypical to suggest possible tumor, biopsy or curettage is indicated.

252

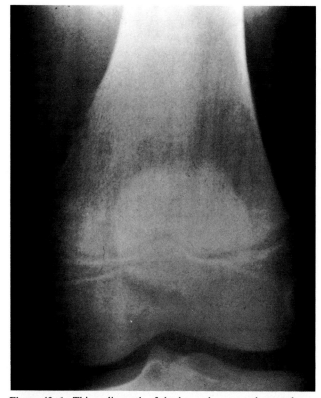

**Figure 43–1.** This radiograph of the knee shows an elongated area of cortical irregularity along the posterior medial cortex. This region is the most common location for an avulsive cortical irregularity.

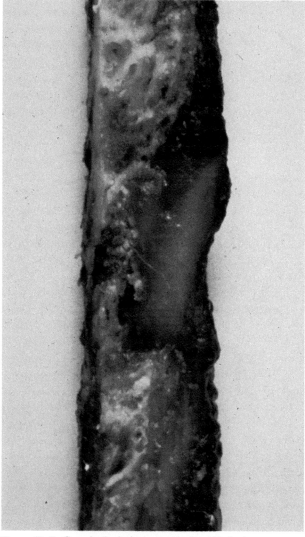

**Figure 43–3.** Grossly the lesion presents the pathologic appearance of a small, nondescript region of fibrous tissue associated with the underlying cortical abnormality.

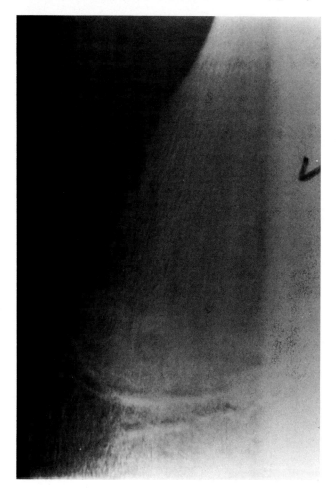

**Figure 43–2.** Closer scrutiny of the region shows spiculation of the posterior medial cortex in the region of the supracondylar ridge. Such avulsive cortical irregularities are nearly always incidental radiographic findings.

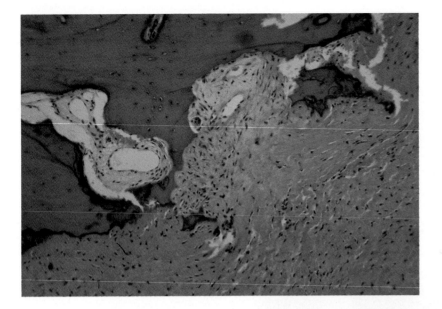

**Figure 43–4.** At low magnification the lesion is composed of spindle cells. The lesion is hypocellular, and abundant collagen production may be present.

**Figure 43–5.** At higher magnification the irregularity of the underlying cortical bone is evident, as this photomicrograph shows. The spindle cells lack cytologic atypia, and the nuclei are uniform, round, and normochromic.

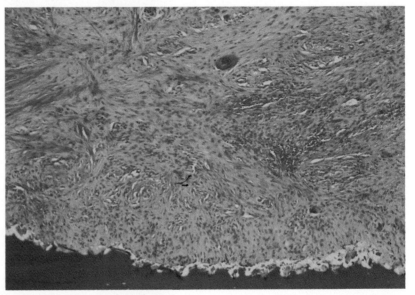

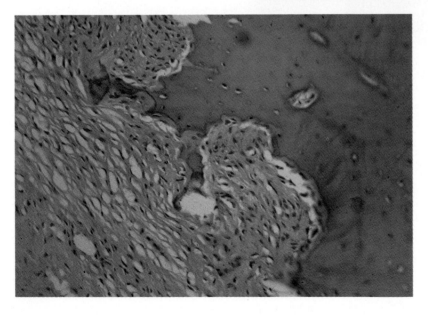

**Figure 43–6.** At high magnification, no mitotic activity is evident and the cytologic features are those of mature fibroblasts.

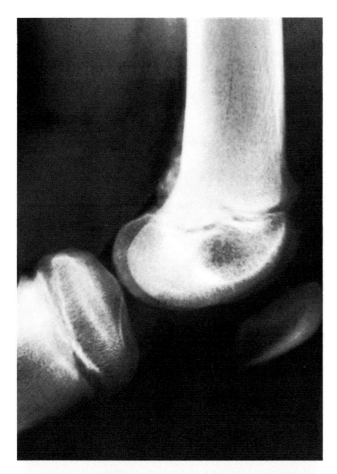

**Figure 43–7.** This lateral radiograph shows an avulsive cortical irregularity of the distal femur with associated new bone formation. Such reactive new bone may alarm the attending physician and raise the suspicion that the lesion represents a malignancy; however, the characteristic location is helpful in correctly identifying the lesion radiographically.

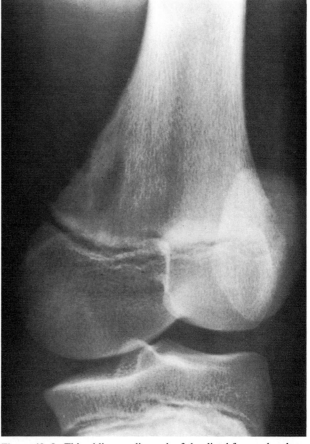

**Figure 43–8.** This oblique radiograph of the distal femur also demonstrates the cortical irregularity of the femur, as well as the lytic defects and fuzzy, irregular cortical surface commonly associated with this condition.

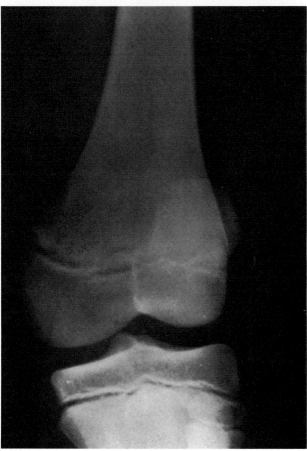

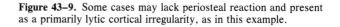

**Figure 43–9.** Some cases may lack periosteal reaction and present as a primarily lytic cortical irregularity, as in this example.

# CHAPTER 44

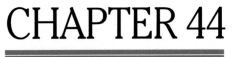

# Hamartoma (Mesenchymoma) of the Chest Wall

*Peak age:*
  Infant years.
*Male to female ratio:*
  Approximately 1 to 1.
*Most common location:*
  Exclusively limited to the chest wall.

■ **Clinical Symptoms**

1. The lesion may be asymptomatic.
2. Difficulty in breathing due to mechanical compromise of the underlying lung may occur.
3. The majority are identified at birth but may not be appreciated until after six months of age.
4. A localized swelling of the chest is usually seen.

■ **Clinical Signs**

1. A mass lesion is present in the chest wall.
2. Respiratory distress, which varies depending upon the size of the lesion, is experienced.

■ **Major Radiographic Features**

1. This is a chest wall lesion of infants.
2. It is often large and usually partially mineralized.
3. One or more ribs are involved, with a combination of erosion and destruction.

■ **Radiographic Differential Diagnosis**

1. Aneurysmal bone cyst.
2. Soft tissue tumor.

■ **Pathologic Features**

*Gross*

1. The lesional tissue is well circumscribed.
2. Cystic blood-filled spaces may make up a significant proportion of the lesional tissue.
3. The lesional tissue is variable in consistency, but fibrous and chondroid regions may be identified.
4. Calcification may be focally present, particularly at the periphery of the lesion.

*Microscopic*

1. At low magnification the lesion varies from region to region.
2. Islands of cartilage resembling epiphyseal plate

are identified within regions of spindled cells.
3. Ossifying trabeculae of bone may be identified in the regions of fibroblastic proliferation.
4. The cystic regions are blood filled and resemble aneurysmal bone cyst.
5. At higher magnification the proliferating cells lack cytologic atypia.
6. Although mitotic activity may be seen, the lesion is well circumscribed and atypical mitoses are not present.

## ■ Pathologic Differential Diagnosis

Benign lesions:
1. Aneurysmal bone cyst.
2. Fibrocartilaginous dysplasia.

Malignant lesions:
1. Osteosarcoma.
2. Fibrosarcoma.

## ■ Treatment

**Primary Modality:** resection with a marginal or wide surgical margin.
**Other Possible Approaches:** may regress without treatment.

## Reference

McLeod RA, and Dahlin DC: Hamartoma (mesenchymoma) of the chest wall in infancy. Radiology *131*:657–661, 1979.

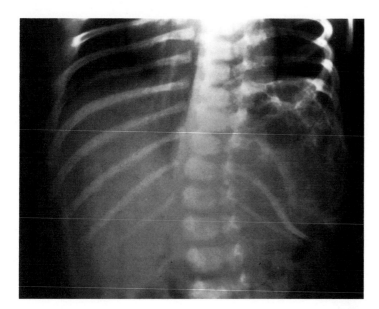

**Figure 44–1.** This radiograph shows a large hamartoma of the wall of the left lower chest. The lesion is irregularly calcified and shows partial destruction of the seventh through tenth ribs.

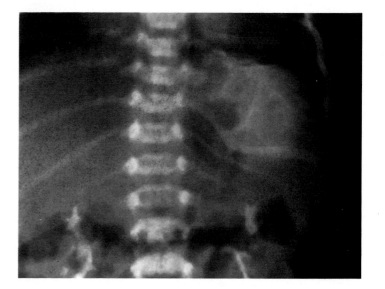

**Figure 44–2.** This radiograph illustrates the features of a hamartoma of the eighth through tenth ribs on the left side.

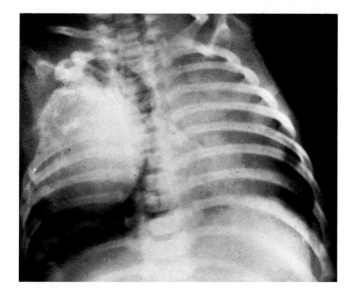

**Figure 44–3.** The size of such hamartomatous lesions is variable. This radiograph shows a very large lesion involving the right upper chest; it contains a small amount of calcification in the upper portion of the soft tissue mass.

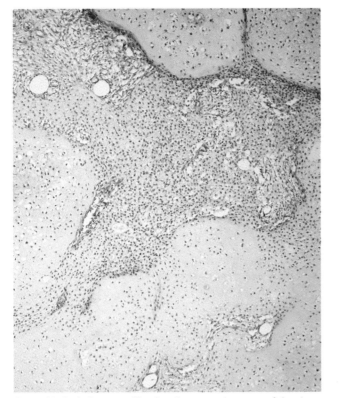

Figure 44–4. At low magnification the mesenchymoma of the chest wall shows a variable histology. Chondroid regions are separated by more cellular regions, as shown in this photomicrograph.

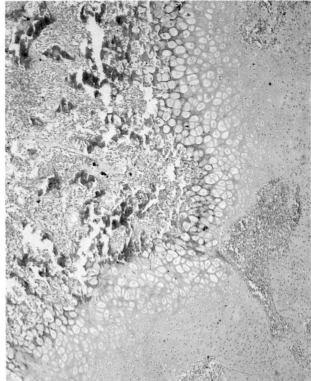

Figure 44–6. This photomicrograph illustrates the juxtaposition of normal cartilage and lesional cartilage in a mesenchymoma of the chest wall in a newborn male.

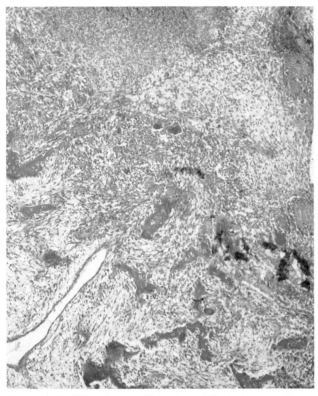

Figure 44–5. Although the solid portions of the lesion may show a worrisome spindle cell proliferation, mature bony trabeculae appear to arise from the spindle cell portion of the lesion, as this photomicrograph shows.

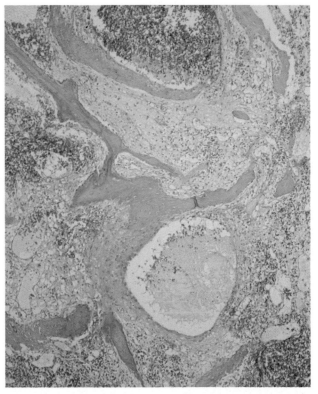

Figure 44–7. Aneurysmal bone cyst–like regions are commonly found in mesenchymomas of the chest wall. Such a region is shown in this photomicrograph.

# CHAPTER 45

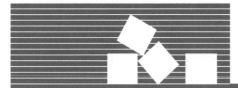

# Osteofibrous Dysplasia

*Peak age:*
    One to five years.
*Male to female ratio:*
    1.5 to 1.
*Most common location:*
    Almost exclusively involves the tibia but may also involve the fibula.

■ **Clinical Symptoms**

1. A swelling of the lower portion of the lower extremity anteriorly is the most common presenting complaint.
2. Anterior or anterolateral bowing of the tibia may be noted.
3. The lesion is usually painless.
4. Sudden pain may be associated with pathologic fracture through the lesion.

■ **Clinical Signs**

1. Bowing of the tibia and fibula is seen.
2. A painless mass lesion overlies the tibia anteriorly.

■ **Major Radiographic Features**

1. The lesion is characteristically located in the tibial diaphysis.
2. Involvement is entirely or predominantly in the cortex, which is often expanded and thinned.
3. Multiple radiolucencies with intervening sclerosis are seen.
4. There is absence of periosteal new bone formation.
5. Bowing of the tibia is evident.

■ **Radiographic Differential Diagnosis**

1. Adamantinoma.
2. Fibrous dysplasia.
3. Nonossifying fibroma.

■ **Pathologic Features**

*Gross*

1. The periosteum overlying the lesion is usually well preserved. The lesion is predominantly cortical.
2. The lesional tissue is generally soft in consistency.
3. A slightly granular quality may be appreciated when the lesional tissue is cut.
4. The color of the lesional tissue varies from whitish-yellow to reddish.

*Microscopic*

1. At low magnification the lesion is composed of hypocellular spindle cells and bony trabeculae.
2. In general, there is prominent osteoblastic rimming of the bony trabeculae.
3. The fibroblastic spindle cell component of the lesion is generally arranged in a loose manner and may show a storiform pattern.

4. Multinucleated giant cells may be identified.
5. At higher magnification the proliferating spindle cells are uniform and lack cytologic atypia.

## ■ Pathologic Differential Diagnosis

Benign lesions:
1. Fibrous dysplasia.
Malignant lesions:
1. Adamantinoma.
2. Low-grade central osteosarcoma.

## ■ Treatment

**Primary Modality:** The lesion shows variable man-ifestations, and observation is indicated if it is asymptomatic.

**Other Possible Approaches:** Surgical excision and bone grafting should be delayed until after age 10, if possible, because of a high incidence of recurrence prior to this age. Osteotomy and internal fixation may be necessary to correct deformities, particularly in the proximal femur.

## References

Campanacci M, and Laus M: Osteofibrous dysplasia of the tibia and fibula. J Bone Joint Surg 63A:367–375, 1981.
Kempson RL: Ossifying fibroma of the long bones: a light and electron microscopic study. Arch Pathol 82:218–233, 1966.

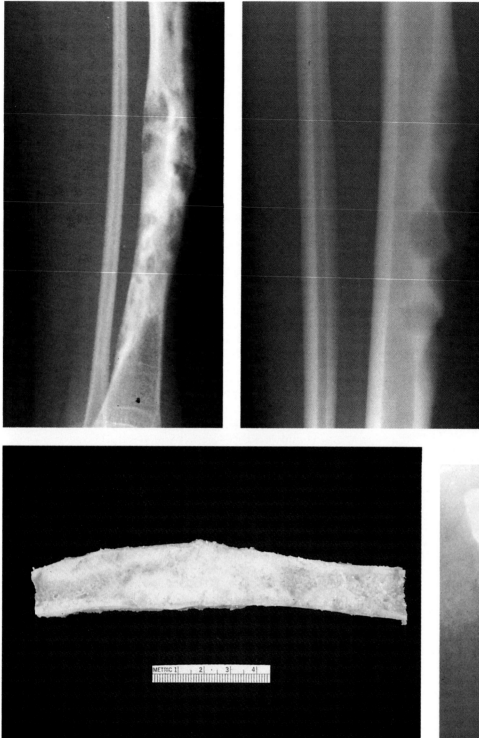

**Figure 45–1.** This radiograph shows osteofibrous dysplasia of the tibial diaphysis. Note the anterior bowing caused by this process, consisting of multiple cortical lucencies with intervening sclerosis.

**Figure 45–3.** This example of osteofibrous dysplasia shows multiple cortical lucencies of the anterior cortex of the midtibia.

**Figure 45–2.** This resected gross specimen corresponds to the radiograph in Figure 45–1. The cortex is thickened, and multiple regions of fibrous connective tissue have resulted in deformation of the bone with resultant bowing of the tibia.

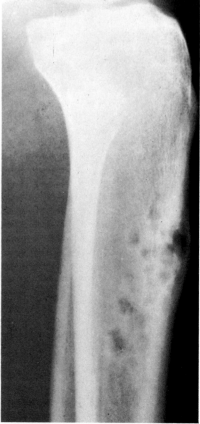

**Figure 45–4.** The cortex may be expanded and thinned in osteofibrous dysplasia, as is illustrated in this radiograph, which also shows multiple cortical lucencies with intervening sclerosis.

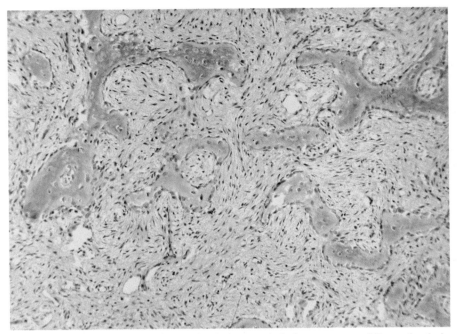

**Figure 45–5.** Histologically osteofibrous dysplasia may mimic the appearance of fibrous dysplasia, as this photomicrograph demonstrates. The bony trabeculae are irregular in shape as in fibrous dysplasia but classically are "rimmed" by prominent osteoblasts, as shown in this example.

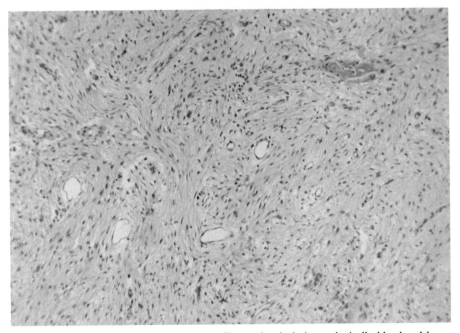

**Figure 45–6.** The fibrous component in osteofibrous dysplasia is cytologically bland and hypocellular. The appearance of this component of the lesion may mimic that of adamantinoma; a careful search for any epithelioid components should be undertaken to exclude the latter diagnosis, since radiographically the lesions may be indistinguishable.

# CHAPTER 46

# Metastatic Carcinoma

*Peak age:*
Adulthood.
*Male to female ratio:*
Approximately 1 to 1.
*Most common location:*
May involve any bone but is rare distal to the elbows and knees.

## ■ Clinical Symptoms

1. Pain is the most common symptom; however, metastatic lesions may be asymptomatic and discovered incidentally on radiographic evaluation for an unrelated problem.
2. Swelling may be noticed in the region of the affected bone.

## ■ Clinical Signs

1. Tenderness is noted in the region of the affected bone.
2. A mass lesion is found.
3. Pathologic fracture is present.

## ■ Major Radiographic Features

1. Solitary or, more commonly, multiple lesions arise centrally in a patient with a known primary malignancy.
2. They are usually detected by combined use of radiographic survey and isotope bone scan.
3. Presentations are diverse, with lytic, blastic, or mixed lesions all common.

## ■ Radiographic Differential Diagnosis

1. Multiple myeloma.
2. Lymphoma.
3. "Brown tumor" of hyperparathyroidism.
4. Many primary malignancies of bone, if solitary.

## ■ Pathologic Features

### Gross

1. The consistency of metastatic lesions varies from firm in those tumors that elicit a desmoplastic stromal reaction to soft in those that do not.
2. The color of the lesions is variable, depending upon the presence or absence of hemorrhage, necrosis, or lipidization of the tumor (as in hypernephroma).
3. The tumors tend to be poorly circumscribed and grow in an invasive, permeative manner.

### Microscopic

1. The majority of carcinomas metastatic to bone show obvious glandular or squamous differentiation at low magnification.
2. If obvious glandular or squamous differentiation is lacking, growth in a clustered or organoid pattern is helpful in identifying the lesion as epithelial in origin.
3. Poorly differentiated carcinomas may grow in a sarcomatous pattern and may consist almost entirely of spindled cells. This is particularly common with renal cell carcinomas.
4. Ultrastructural and immunohistochemical investigation of sarcomatous malignancies in patients over 60 years of age without predisposing factors

for developing a primary sarcoma (e.g., Paget's disease, prior radiation, etc.) may show epithelial characteristics.

### ■ Pathologic Differential Diagnosis

Malignant lesions:
1. Fibrosarcoma.
2. Malignant fibrous histiocytoma.

### ■ Treatment

**Primary Modality:** requires multidisciplinary team approach that includes (1) careful attention to the patient's general health and correction of nutritional and metabolic problems; (2) aggressive systemic treatment to control the basic neoplastic process; and (3) the use of radiation therapy as the primary modality to control local symptoms, which provides effective pain relief for up to one year in 80 per cent of patients.

**Other Possible Approaches:** internal fixation or prosthetic replacement for actual or imminent pathologic fractures.

### References

Fitzgerald RH Jr, Brewer NS, and Dahlin DC: Squamous-cell carcinoma complicating chronic osteomyelitis. J Bone Joint Surg 58A:1146–1148, 1976.

Sim FH (ed): Diagnosis and Treatment of Metastatic Bone Disease: A Multidisciplinary Approach to Management. New York: Raven Press, 1987.

Simon MA, and Karluk MB: Skeletal metastases of unknown origin: diagnostic strategy for orthopedic surgeons. Clin Orthop 166:96–103, 1982.

Tomera KM, Farrow GM, and Lieber MM: Sarcomatoid renal carcinoma. J Urol 130:657–659, 1983.

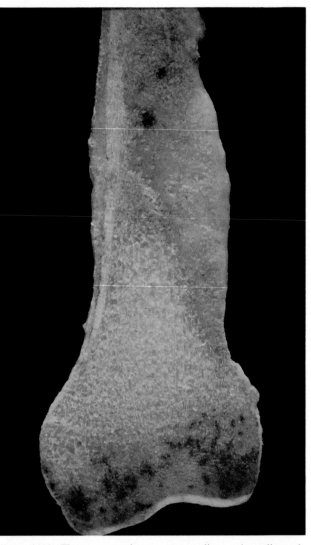

**Figure 46–2.** The gross specimen corresponding to the radiograph in Figure 46–1 shows a destructive diametaphyseal tumor with diaphyseal cortical destruction. The tumor is firm, white, and fibrous.

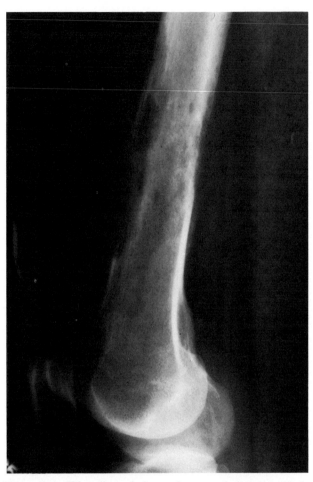

**Figure 46–1.** This radiograph shows a large, poorly marginated lytic lesion of the lower diametaphyseal region of the lower femur. This elderly male patient had a known carcinoma of the lung.

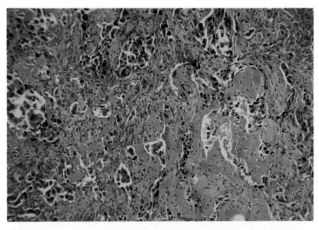

**Figure 46–3.** At low magnification metastatic adenocarcinomas generally can be seen to show gland formation, as this photomicrograph illustrates. An osteoblastic response by the bone, if it is pronounced, may obscure the metastatic tumor.

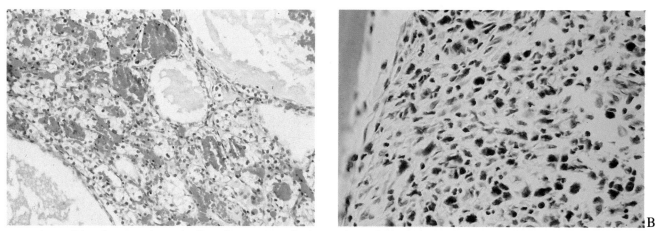

**Figure 46–4.** Although metastatic renal cell carcinomas generally show a clear cell histologic pattern of differentiation (*A*), metastases from a sarcomatoid renal cell carcinoma may mimic a primary bone tumor (*B*). Fortunately, in general there will be a history of a preceding renal malignancy.

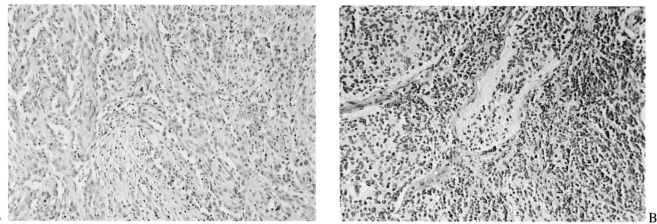

**Figure 46–5.** *A* shows a metastatic papillary carcinoma that in some areas grew in a pattern mimicking that of a vascular tumor. Although uncommon, metastatic neuroblastoma (*B*) can mimic a "small blue cell tumor" if rosettes and neuropil are not recognized.

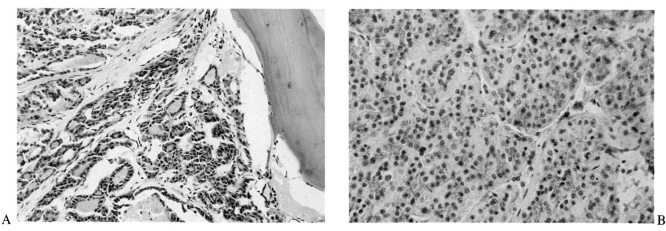

**Figure 46–6.** At times it may be possible to suggest a site of origin of an osseous metastasis on the basis of its histologic pattern of growth. *A* shows a metastatic follicular carcinoma of the thyroid; *B* illustrates a metastatic hepatocellular carcinoma in which bile could be seen.

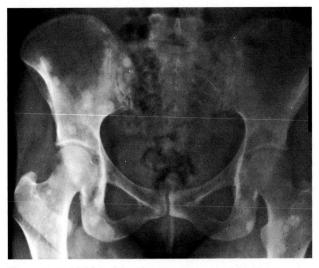

**Figure 46–7.** Multiple sclerotic metastases are visible in the pelvis of this elderly female with a prior diagnosis of carcinoma of the breast.

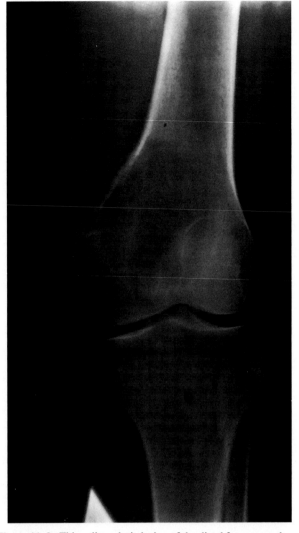

**Figure 46–8.** This solitary lytic lesion of the distal femur was shown to represent metastatic renal cell carcinoma on biopsy. In this location a giant cell tumor could also be considered in the differential diagnosis.

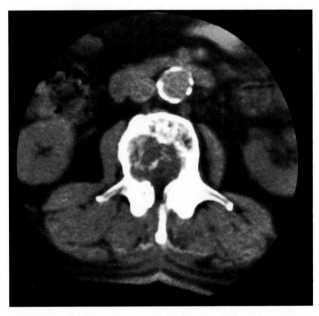

**Figure 46–9.** A CT scan may be helpful in identifying metastasis, as is demonstrated by this view showing a mixed lytic and sclerotic metastasis in the lumbar vertebra.

# INDEX

Note: Page numbers in *italics* refer to illustrations.